Confident Choices

Customizing the Interstitial Cystitis Diet

Julie Beyer, RD
NutraConsults, LLC

Copyright © 2005 Julie Beyer, RD
All Rights Reserved

No part of this book may be used or reproduced in any manner without written permission except on pages designated for reproduction and in brief quotations in critical articles and reviews.

Published in the United States of America by:

NutraConsults, LLC
P.O. Box 210086, Auburn Hills, MI 48321
www.NutraConsults.com

ISBN 0-9767246-0-X

To order a copy of this book, please visit:
www.NutraConsults.com/confidentchoices.html

Disclaimer: Confident Choices, a division of NutraConsults, LLC, is not a medical authority. No information written or implied in this workbook, the Confident Choices' website, or the Confident Choices' newsletter, or any resource recommended should be considered medical advice. Please contact your physician for information regarding any change you wish to make in your lifestyle. Confident Choices urges you to carefully research ANY information that you find regarding health and wellness, including information received from NutraConsults.

Trademark notice: This book uses various trademarked names within its text. In the interest of the reader, we are using the trademarked names in an editorial style. In the interest of the trademark holders, we cite their ownership of the trademarks, with no intention of infringement.

Time sensitive materials: At the time of publication, all names, addresses, telephone numbers, email and Web addresses were verified as accurate.

Dedications

To the IC patients who selflessly nurtured me when I was first diagnosed: Yvette, Lesa, Donna, Martha, Rachel, Teri, Jane, Dede, and our IC Angel Diane, I continue to be humbled by your dedication, love, and support.

To the people who, by their quiet example, first taught me to care for others. Mom and Dad, I miss you every moment of every day.

Special Thanks

Life doesn't stop when you write a book. Someone has to cook, wash the dishes, do the laundry, and water the plants while the mommy hides in her office and writes:

Jim, Rebekah, Carolyn, and Daniel,

without your support, this book never would have made it to print. I can't express how much I love you and how proud I am of you. Let's go to Disney World.

Also.........

To Jill Osborn, founder of the Interstitial Cystitis Network: Thank you for sharing your wisdom. Because of you, I didn't have to start from scratch.

To Holly Helterhoff, my editor: Thank you for your patient genius and for rescuing me from all those exclamation marks! YOU are the Rock Star!

To Gita Patel MS RD CDE LD: Thank you for critically reviewing the book from the dietitian's point of view. Your last minute encouragement was priceless.

To everyone who squeezed time out of their busy schedules to proofread the manuscript: Jim, Rebekah, and Carolyn Beyer, Lesa Ferenz, Myria Johnson, Peter Johnson, Rachel Newman, Katrina Spaeth, Martha Steinman, and Kim VanMeter

Contents

	Introduction	1
1.	An Interstitial Cystitis Primer	7
2.	Understanding IC and Diet	15
3.	Food for Flares	20
4.	Discovering Your Personal Trigger Foods	27
	a. Voiding and Pain Diary	37
	b. Food Intake Diary	38
	c. IC Food List	39
	d. Sample Pain Level	43
	e. Sample Grocery List	44
5.	Planning Meals	49
6.	Breakfast	58
7.	Lunch	63
8.	Dinner	70
9.	Beverages	75
10.	Recipes	83
11.	Dietary Supplements for IC	107
12.	Exercise and Fitness	117
13.	Making Peace with Stress	126
14.	IC Diet Success Stories	135
15.	Resources	145

Introduction

*"The best effect of any book
is that it excites the reader to self-activity."*
Thomas Carlyle

Before We Begin

It is likely you bought this book because you either have interstitial cystitis (IC), you suspect you do, or someone you care about has it. I imagine some health care professionals will read this book also. The commonality is, if you have this book in your hands, you already know something about interstitial cystitis.

What you may not know is that IC terminology is changing in some medical circles, and IC is likely to be called something different in a few years. The idea is to be more inclusive of other syndromes that are similar to IC. Men might currently be diagnosed with "non-bacterial prostatitis," yet their symptoms respond to classic IC treatments. Or, maybe you were diagnosed with Chronic Pelvic Pain Syndrome (CPPS) or Painful Bladder Syndrome (PBS). For simplicity, this printing of *Confident Choices* will use the terms "interstitial cystitis" or "IC" to encompass all of the above conditions. As *Confident*

Choices is revised, the terminology may change. The process of individualizing your diet is the same.

You may also wonder, "Where is the research to support dietary modification as a treatment for interstitial cystitis?" The answer is simple: there isn't much research, but hopefully there will be in the near future. In the meantime, there is ample anecdotal evidence that dietary modification can be a successful addition to a patient's comprehensive treatment plan. In fact, over 91% of patients who responded to a February 2004 online survey done by the Interstitial Cystitis Association (www.ichelp.org) reported that certain foods or beverages make their symptoms worse, and over 84% of those patients reported some symptom relief by modifying their diet. I do not know of any other therapy for IC that can boast those numbers.

Over time, physicians and patients who noticed this dietary connection distributed an assortment of "good food/bad food" lists. Although you might be confused by the differences of the various lists, any IC diet list should only be used as a foundation for individualized dietary modification. The purpose of learning to apply the elimination diet techniques discussed in this book is to create a personalized list of safe foods and trigger foods. *Confident Choices* begins by using a modified version of the IC Diet found on the Interstitial Cystitis Network (www.ic-network.com).

Be Persistent

Sometimes, while trying to modify your diet, it may seem that your symptoms are not improving. Since many factors can influence the intensity of IC symptoms (medications, activities, stress, even lack of sleep), sometimes dietary modification effects can be masked. If at any time you feel this is happening, I would like to encourage you to try the elimination techniques again at a later date.

Perhaps you are one of the many IC patients who has been diagnosed with other conditions that require dietary modification such as diabetes or heart disease. Since it is impossible to include every conceivable combination diet scenario in this book, I advise you to seek the counsel of a registered dietitian (RD). RDs are medical professionals who are experts in dietary modification and medical nutrition therapy. To find an RD near you, visit the American Dietetic Association at www.eatright.org and use the search feature entitled "Find a Nutrition Professional." You can also email me at NutraConsults@aol.com, and I will help you locate someone.

Beyond Diet

Another fascinating area related to IC and diet is the use of complementary and alternative medicine (CAM) therapies. Many researchers are examining the use of nutritional supplements, various herbs, and other natural substances as adjuncts in IC therapies. Although many compounds are showing promise as possible treatments for IC, it is important to remember that science is generally a very slow process. Keep in mind that information about alternative medicines or nutritional supplements is likely to change repeatedly as doctors and scientists perform more studies and refine their research techniques. Although this book contains information about some common alternative medicine supplements, please remember that every patient is an individual, and recommendations for supplements should come solely through your personal physician. This communication is vital for you to know that your other treatments are not compromised or the results disguised. On the other hand, if a supplement does work for you, that knowledge may help your physician help other IC patients.

Obviously, modifying your diet is not the only way to improve your health and sense of well-being. Increasing your physical activity and practicing stress reduction techniques can potentially reduce the severity of IC symptoms and can give you a sense of control in a situation that often seems out of control.

> *There is nothing so moving, not even acts of love or hate, as the discovery that one is not alone."*
> Robert Ardrey
> The Interstitial Cystitis Network Motto

One of the best ways to adjust to having a chronic illness like IC is to meet other people who are learning to cope with a similar condition. IC patients who participate in local or online support groups generally express a higher level of well-being than patients who do not have support. Not only do patients benefit from sharing coping strategies with each other, but also, many support groups invite leading IC researchers and physicians to share the latest information about treatments.

Sorting Out Research

One of the first things most people do after being diagnosed with a chronic illness is research all that they can about the disease. Now, as a dietitian and health educator, I have resources available to me that guide me in sorting out the facts of medical research, but what about everyone else? The sciences of medicine and nutrition often look chaotic to average consumers, who must sort through exaggerated reports, sketchy claims, and even genuine scientific progress that may contradict previous knowledge. It is no wonder that many people become cynical.

So, how can you determine if medical research is valid and applicable to you?

1. Check the credibility of the journal publishing the study. Are articles reviewed by other researchers before publication?

2. What is the stated objective of the study? Is it clearly defined or vague? Non-specific objectives may lead to flawed conclusions.

3. Was the study based on reliable formative research? Rarely does a study stand alone. Someone discovered something about the topic before it was studied in the current form. When you compare the results to previous studies, is there some logical progression of new knowledge formed?

4. How many people were in the study? How was the population chosen for study? Was it a random sample of people? Were concrete parameters designed to help ensure randomization of test and control groups? Randomization of study subjects helps ensure more significant results.

5. Do the researchers suggest further related studies? Quality research always acknowledges that it is only a part of the puzzle.

6. Does the discussion of the study discuss flaws inherent in the study design? This is actually a good thing to know. Honest and reliable researchers are not afraid to talk about where they may have gone wrong.

Now, where do you FIND research articles? Many junior or community colleges allow the citizens of their community access to their academic databases even if they are not students. Online sources may or may not require a membership in an organization, but many do allow limited access to their journal articles. Thankfully, a growing number of organizations post studies and results pertinent to their topic. For example, both the Interstitial Cystitis Network and the Interstitial Cystitis Association have extensive sections on research.

Finally, there is a newly formed resource that brings research results directly to the consumer. A growing number of respected scientific and medical journals are contributing articles to "PatientInform.org," providing previously inaccessible information to consumers.

How to use *Confident Choices*

I suggest that you read or at least skim this whole book before beginning to sort out your trigger foods. You will be more confident if you know in advance where the various charts, diaries, meal plans and recipes are located.

Since you will likely reevaluate your diet on and off for the rest of your life, *Confident Choices* not only provides you with information about IC and diet, but also includes questions at the end of each chapter that are intended to stimulate your own thoughts about the topic. You can either record your thoughts in the spaces provided, or you can keep a separate, personal journal. Although it might be tempting to skip this step, the more ways that you can reinforce what you are learning, the easier it will be to maintain the diet changes and develop the intuition necessary to truly take control of your IC symptoms!

1

An Interstitial Cystitis Primer

"The best way to become acquainted with a subject is to write a book about it."
Benjamin Disraeli

What is Wrong with Me?

I sometimes wonder how many registered dietitians become experts in specific areas of nutrition because a disease or condition has affected their family, friends, or them personally. Certainly, I never sought to become an expert on interstitial cystitis. In fact, I would not claim to be an expert now. Yet in July 1998, after spending years searching for an answer to the cluster of symptoms I was experiencing, my urologist diagnosed me with interstitial cystitis. My reaction to the news was that of a classic IC patient. I was relieved to know what was causing my pain, but the diagnosis itself was still a shock. All I knew about IC at the time was that you had to follow a special diet, and that the disease never went away.

In the months following my diagnosis, my urologist and his nurse patiently answered all of my questions, and I searched the Internet for any information I could find about this puzzling disease. At the time there were only a few books published that addressed interstitial cystitis. Many references described "cystitis" in terms of a urinary tract infection. Although symptoms of IC can feel like a urinary tract infection, the condition is sterile. I began describing it to people as the difference between a cold and allergies. You may sneeze and get a stuffy nose with both conditions, but a cold is caused by a germ, and allergies are not.

Symptoms of IC

The most common symptoms of IC include:

- Urinary frequency (commonly 20+ times/day)
- Nocturia (the need to wake several times in the night to urinate)
- Urgency (an insistent and immediate need to urinate)
- Dyspareunia (painful intercourse)
- Lower abdominal pressure and/or pain

An estimated 700,000 people, in the US have been diagnosed with IC This number is expected to exceed one million as more physicians become aware of IC, diagnostic techniques improve, and diagnostic criteria are modified to reflect current knowledge of the disease. Approximately 90% of IC patients are women, and at this time, there is no identifiable cause (such as a bacterial infection). Some patients report experiencing stressful events, frequent urinary tract infections, or some sort of pelvic injury just prior to the onset of symptoms, any of which could damage the bladder lining, producing the cluster of symptoms familiar to IC patients.

Diagnosis

As you may have experienced, the path to being diagnosed with IC can be frustrating. Physicians may take months or years to rule out other urinary tract diseases such as infection or cancer. Patients are likely to seek the help of multiple practitioners before a definitive diagnosis is made. Examination of the bladder wall by cystoscopy, generally done under anesthesia, often reveals inflammation, damage to the bladder lining, and/or wounds in the bladder. This procedure could also reveal increased mast cells, which are involved in immune system functions and inflammatory processes. The urologist may also perform a procedure called a hydrodistention in which the bladder is filled with a sterile liquid and "stretched," offering the urologist a different view of the bladder lining. Sometimes, a hydrodistention temporarily relieves the patient's symptoms, thus, it is occasionally used as a treatment for IC. Once in awhile, the bladders of patients do not show these visible signs, and a diagnosis is based solely on clinical symptoms and patient history.

More recently, physicians have used a potassium instillation (filling the bladder with a potassium solution) as a diagnostic tool. If the bladder wall is damaged, the potassium solution will be very painful for the patient, and the diagnosis of IC is highly likely. A rescue solution of lidocaine is used to immediately numb the bladder and reduce the patient's discomfort. Although this procedure sounds archaic to some, it does not require outpatient surgery under anesthesia, and the recovery time is minimal.

The ideal situation, however, would be to have a simple urine test that identifies some substance in the urine of IC patients that differs from those without IC. That possibility may become a typical diagnostic event in the near future. Susan Keay, M.D. and others from the University of Maryland School of Medicine have identified such a substance in the urine of IC patients called the antiproliferative factor (APF). APF is made specifically by bladder epithelial cells in patients with IC. This APF seems to keep the bladder cells from reproducing properly and may also be a clue to the cause of some cases of IC.

Treatment Options for IC

At this time, treatments are available to reduce symptoms, improve quality of life, and possibly provide relief in the form of a remission, but there is no "cure" for IC. Treatment plans are individualized for each patient, and with patience, a temporary remission can be achieved by combining lifestyle changes, medications, and dietary modification. Medical treatments are often experimental and may take months of trials before seeing if there will be any benefits.

Oral medications are available to treat various symptoms. The only oral medication approved specifically for use as a treatment for IC is Elmiron (pentosan polysulfate sodium). Elmiron appears to improve the protective qualities of the bladder lining. Oral medications used to treat pain in IC patients include urinary anesthetics (Pyridium and Uristat), tri-cyclic antidepressants, opiates, and anti-inflammatory agents. Various antihistamines (hydroxyzine HCL or hydroxyzine pomoate) can be used successfully to reduce symptoms in patients who have demonstrated high mast cell distribution. Antihistamines can also reduce anxiety and act as a sleep aid for IC patients. Urinary anti-spasmodics (Ditropan and Detrol) are sometimes prescribed for IC patients, but generally do not control all of the symptoms. Antibiotic and antifungal therapy are controversial as treatments, but may be considered if an infection is suspected despite sterile urine cultures.

Other medical treatments include hydrodistention, surgical removal of ulcerated or scarred bladder tissue, and as a last resort, removal of the bladder. Various medications, instilled directly into the bladder can be helpful for some patients. External and internal electrical stimulation devices have been used successfully in some patients, although overall results have been mixed. Allergy testing and treatment may seem like an unusual therapy for IC, but some patients report a decrease in their symptoms when they undergo allergy treatment.

Luckily, diet and lifestyle modifications along with other coping strategies are often highly successful for IC patients. It is very important for IC patients to get adequate sleep and learn relaxation techniques such as stretching exercises, yoga, biofeedback, or deep breathing. Many patients and their partners find that with patience, sexual activity can still be an important and fulfilling part of their lives. And of course, counselors can provide a stable link in treatment for the IC patient, helping them learn to cope with a chronic illness and guiding them through the often lengthy and frustrating process of finding a combination of treatments that work.

The Journey to Acceptance

Being diagnosed with a chronic illness is not in anyone's life plan. Not only do you have to adjust to the concept of being ill, but negotiating treatments and lifestyle changes can leave you flooding with emotions, interfering with your efforts to get well. Indeed, if you have been diagnosed with IC, you can expect to go through several predictable stages: denial, anger, depression, bargaining and finally acceptance. It is important to recognize that friends and family members may also experience the various stages of grief and acceptance.

Try to keep the stages in mind as you explore how foods can trigger your IC symptoms. Most likely you will have times of denial, anger, and depression as you figure out your diet. Most people don't pass through these stages in order. Instead, they bounce back and forth between stages as they face different challenges along the way. To successfully navigate the stages of acceptance, you need to learn as much as you can about your illness and develop a "take control" attitude.

So now it is your turn. Take some time to reflect on your experiences with IC, its symptoms and diagnostic procedures. Is your story similar to others you have heard? What makes your situation unique?

Taking Control:

Have you been diagnosed with IC or a similar bladder condition? If so, how long ago were you diagnosed?

_____
_____

How many physicians did you see before you were diagnosed? What is your diagnosis "story?"

_____
_____
_____
_____
_____
_____

How would you describe your IC symptoms?

_____
_____
_____
_____
_____
_____

Do you believe that your symptoms disrupt or change your daily life in any way? If so, how?

_____
_____
_____
_____
_____
_____
_____

Do you believe that your symptoms have disrupted or changed any of your personal or family relationships? If your symptoms do disrupt your relationships, what has changed?

_____
_____
_____
_____
_____
_____
_____
_____
_____

What treatments and/or medications have you tried (both before and after diagnosis)? What was your experience with each?

_____
_____
_____
_____
_____
_____
_____
_____
_____

What treatments and/or medications are you using right now? How would you rate the effectiveness of your current treatments/medications?

_____
_____
_____
_____
_____
_____

What coping strategies do you use to help keep your IC symptoms under control?

_____
_____
_____
_____
_____
_____
_____
_____
_____

2

Understanding IC and Diet

"Science seldom proceeds in the straightforward logical manner imagined by outsiders. Instead, its steps forward (and sometimes backward) are often very human events in which personalities and cultural traditions play major roles."
James Watson in *The Double Helix*, a book recounting his experience discovering the structure of DNA

Is There an IC Diet?

When first diagnosed, I was not that intimidated by the IC dietary restrictions. I felt certain that I could successfully navigate meals by faithfully following the food list provided by my urologist's nurse. But later that summer, at an event where lunch was being served, my confidence faded. The only food offered was pepperoni pizza, and drinks were limited to beer and carbonated beverages. I realized that there was nothing offered that I could eat or drink. Instantly, I realized that my relationship with food had changed forever.

Like many IC patients, I initially believed that the IC diet was a good food/bad food list that needed to be followed strictly. But after that luncheon, I began to dig deeper into the origin of such a restrictive diet. Surprisingly, I found that very little clinical research had been done to determine the effects of diet in IC patients. For a while, I even used this fact as rationale for *not* modifying my diet. As you can guess, my symptoms didn't improve for a long time.

I did find that, despite the lack of scientific evidence linking diet to IC, the effects of particular foods on interstitial cystitis symptoms have been observed by patients and doctors for decades. As a result, various forms of the "IC Diet" have been distributed over the past 20 years. Foods such as coffee, tea, sodas, alcoholic beverages, artificial sweeteners, tomatoes, strawberries, citrus fruits, and soy are frequently cited as triggers for IC symptoms. In fact, cranberry juice, often used as a natural remedy for bacterial urinary tract infections, is considered to be one of the worst offenders for IC.

How Does Diet Affect IC Symptoms?

There is no indication that any food or food group causes IC. Researchers do have many theories about how and why certain foods affect IC symptoms. Because specific foods can affect individual IC patients differently, some believe there may be an allergy component. Other foods, such as caffeinated products, MSG, and spices, may be chemical or physiological irritants. For those IC patients who don't believe that food makes a difference in their IC, remember that foods can affect all of the symptoms of IC. You may not experience an increase in pain, but you may have an increase in frequency or urgency.

Some IC patients attempt to avoid all acidic foods because many of the common trigger foods are acidic in nature. The problem with this theory is that foods and beverages are digested differently, and an acidic food may not contribute to acidic urine. Citrus fruits, for example, cause urine to become slightly more alkaline, whereas cranberry juice can slightly acidify the urine. Both foods are considered common bladder irritants in IC patients. For people with healthy bladders, this variation in urine pH is not even noticeable. However, if the pH in urine is too low or too high when a person has wounds in their bladder, or their protective bladder lining is defective, the pain can be excruciating.

An area that needs more attention from researchers is how eating an IC friendly diet can potentially affect the outcomes of other medical treatments. It only makes sense that if you are trying to rebuild the bladder lining that you would want to make the bladder environment as hospitable to healing as possible. I believe that one way to accomplish this by reducing the intake of foods that assault the bladder.

On a final note, you may be aware that the current trend in health care is "evidence-based medicine." Consequently, until we learn more about how diet affects IC, you may come across some physicians and dietitians who express skepticism about prescribing dietary modification for IC patients. Unfortunately, that is a bit like the cyclical chicken and the egg story; there isn't any evidence to support an "IC Diet" because no significant research has been done. In the meantime, countless IC patients have successfully improved their condition by changing the foods that they eat. I believe that if something as simple as diet modification has the potential to reduce the severity of IC symptoms, then those of us in the medical community have an obligation to tell patients about it.

Taking Control:

Before now, have you heard about an "IC Diet?" If so, where did you first hear about it?

_____
_____
_____
_____
_____

Do you find that food choices can affect your IC symptoms? If so, which foods do you feel cause you the most problems?

_____
_____
_____
_____
_____
_____
_____

Have you previously tried to modify your diet to control your IC symptoms? If so, what was your experience?

_____
_____
_____
_____
_____
_____
_____
_____
_____

How would you describe your level of motivation and willingness to alter your diet in order to reduce your IC symptoms?

_____
_____
_____
_____

What might affect your success in managing your IC symptoms with diet? (Examples: family support, travel or business obligations, frequently dining out, other dietary restrictions, fear of failure, etc.)

_____
_____
_____
_____
_____
_____
_____
_____

3

Food for Flares

"Always remember, there is more strength in you than you ever realized or even imagined. Certainly nothing can keep you down if you are determined to get on top of things and stay there."
                              Norman Vincent Peale

What is a Flare?

An IC flare is the intense return of IC symptoms in a patient who has been relatively pain free. Symptoms of a flare can include urinary frequency, urgency, and pain. Patients in a flare may also experience extreme fatigue, anxiety and depression as they struggle to cope with the recurrence of symptoms they thought were under control.

Sometimes flares can dissipate in a day, or they may continue on for months at a time. Many times an IC patient will believe that they have a urinary tract infection (UTI), only to find that their urine sample is sterile (I often say that people with IC are the only people who are happy when a urinalysis shows they have a UTI—because they can do something about it!).

Examples of things that can precipitate a flare are certain foods, sexual intercourse, constipation, diarrhea, restrictive clothing, pre-menstrual syndrome, heavy exercise, and stress. Unfortunately, it is not always easy to determine what causes a flare.

IC Rescue Diet

If certain foods can trigger your symptoms, it only makes sense that you should choose bladder safe foods if you are in a flare. The very safest foods include plain chicken, pears, green beans, carrots, rice, distilled or filtered water, milk, eggs, and white bread products. Since flares are unpredictable, it is also wise to keep these foods on hand. Keep chicken, green beans, and white bread in the freezer to pull out at the last minute. Pears and carrots can be canned. Rice can be instant or long grain. (I love using a rice maker. In twenty minutes we have the base for almost any meal!)

You should see positive results within three days of following this very minimal "rescue" diet. Please note that this diet is nutritionally deficient, and should not be consumed for longer than a week. If you do not experience relief after a few days, I recommend that you contact your physician. If your physician says that you need to follow this minimal diet longer than a week, a registered dietitian can help you choose foods to maximize your nutritional intake.

Sample Rescue Menus

When you are in a flare, you may not have the energy to think about what you should eat. It is also very easy to console yourself with comfort foods, some of which may not be the best foods to eat for your condition. Because of that, I have included some sample meal plans to get you started:

Breakfast:
>Scrambled eggs and toast with butter
>Pears
>Milk

Lunch:
>Chicken sandwich with white bread and butter or margarine
>Carrots
>Pears
>Milk

Choose a Snack:
>Bagel
>Toast
>Hard-boiled egg
>Carrots
>Pears
>Milk

Dinner:
>Chicken
>Rice
>Green beans
>Pears
>Milk

Other Self-Help Strategies

Although this book is focused specifically on diet, there are some other things you can do to minimize a flare. If you are constipated or have diarrhea, other dietary adjustments may be more appropriate than the rescue diet provided. Drinking more water and adding fiber are simple self-care ways to correct these problems. If intestinal problems persist, ask your physician for other treatment recommendations.

Other flare management techniques include: getting plenty of rest, practicing stress reduction strategies, taking warm baths with Epsom salts or baking soda, writing in your journal, and talking to other IC patients. You may also find relief from using a heating pad, hot water bottle, or one of those heat pads that stick on the outside of your underwear. Heat can fool the body into thinking that you are not feeling any pelvic pain. Your doctor can also advise you about medications you can use specifically for a flare.

You will probably be more comfortable if you wear loose clothing when you have a flare. Medical scrubs, pajama pants, and sweat pants with adjustable waistbands are good choices. Women may also be more comfortable in jumpers or loose sundresses. Flat shoes or slippers are easier on your back than those with heels.

Sometimes when you have a flare it is hard to think past the pain. To simplify the coping process, you might want to create a list of things to do when you get a flare. Include your urologist's phone number, sample menus, a list of medicines to take, and remind yourself to rest.

Finally, enlist the help of your loved ones. If you prefer not to talk about your illness all the time, decide on a secret phrase to use with your family and friends that signals to them you have an angry bladder. Even small children can understand that your tummy hurts, and most will be content to cuddle on the couch with you and do quiet things.

Flare Coping References

There are dozens of flare coping strategies that are not covered in this chapter. Since finding ways to cope with flares often means trial and error, the best way to learn is to talk to other IC patients at either local support groups or ask questions in an online support group community like the Interstitial

Cystitis Network (www.ic-network.com/forum/). Both the ICN and the ICA have information on IC support groups in your area.

You will probably want to read everything you can about flare management strategy. Please be careful when choosing books about IC or any other health problem. Avoid anything that promises a cure or suggests using any non-documented therapies. A good place to check for a book's credibility is on the websites for the Interstitial Cystitis Association (www.ichelp.org) or the Interstitial Cystitis Network (www.ic-network.com). If the book is not sold or recommended by those organizations, it is probably not worth your money. Several references are discussed in the Resources chapter at the end of the book.

When to Contact your Doctor

Shortly after I was diagnosed with IC, my husband and I drove from Michigan to Florida with our three children, about a twenty-hour drive. I was feeling worse than usual, but I assumed that it was my bladder flaring. Instead of calling the doctor, I took some medicine and tried to enjoy the drive. My symptoms steadily got worse and riding in the van became nearly impossible, I finally asked my husband to stop at an emergency room in north Florida. The doctor said I had the worst urinary tract infection he had ever seen! Thankfully, after 24 hours on antibiotics, I felt great and was able to fully enjoy our vacation.

The lesson is to always call your doctor when you have questions about your symptoms. In fact, there are some red flag symptoms that should be dealt with by calling your physician immediately:

- Severe pain that is not controlled by your normal medications
- Pain or frequency that is *different* than your usual symptoms
- Fever or chills

- Difficulty urinating
- Blood in the urine
- Cloudy or foul smelling urine

Recovering From a Flare

Regardless of which coping strategies you use to get your bladder under control, it is important not to overdo it when you feel better. It may be tempting to work overtime as you catch up on chores and work, but I really believe it is important to rest and eat only the most bladder friendly foods for a week or so after you recover.

Also, try to think about what may have caused the flare in the first place and add these thoughts to your journal. Did you wear restrictive clothing or try a new food? Were you under more stress than usual, or were you not getting enough sleep? By scrutinizing the things that may have caused you to flare, you can minimize your chances for another one!

Taking Control

What are your flare management strategies?

_____
_____
_____
_____
_____
_____
_____
_____
_____

What foods can you have on hand to help you in a flare?

_____
_____
_____
_____
_____
_____
_____
_____

What things can your family or friends do to help you when you are in a flare?

_____
_____
_____
_____
_____
_____
_____
_____
_____

4

Discovering Your Personal Trigger Foods

"Changing our diet is something we choose to do, not something we are forced to do. Instead of dreading it, try saying, "There's another thing I get to do to help myself. Great!"
Greg Anderson, athlete and cancer survivor in
"The 22 Non-Negotiable Laws of Wellness"

It's Personal

I love the lesson of Greg Anderson's life. After being diagnosed with terminal cancer in 1984, Anderson defied his 30-day death sentence and resolutely decided to live. Twenty years later, he is an inspiring speaker and writer who challenges people to take charge of their health and personal well-being by changing the things that are within their power.

If you have been diagnosed with IC, you might feel as though all of the decisions about your life have been placed in someone else's hands. Yet, dietary modification is entirely within your control and can be one of the most successful ways to manage your IC symptoms.

You probably already suspect that certain foods trigger your symptoms. For most IC patients, the worst offenders are tomato products, cranberry juice, citrus fruits, soy, coffee, tea, sodas, alcoholic beverages, and chocolate. Some day we will understand what is happening when an IC patient eats certain foods, but at this point, it doesn't matter. You want to feel better now. If a food is causing you to flare, you don't want to eat it.

Now, it may seem obvious to most people that if something hurts you, you don't do it. That is the physical message that pain is supposed to give us. For example, if you put your hand too close to a flame and get burned, or if you miss a nail and hit your thumb with a hammer, those are lessons you learn almost instantly. There can be many reasons, however, why we resist changing our diet, even though we know we should.

First of all, we have to be convinced that one food or another is causing us difficulty. Sorting it out can seem impossible, so we might not even try. Second, it is easy to deny that particular foods bother us when the foods themselves "mean" so much to us. Look at people's attachments to coffee, chocolate, or sodas. In some ways we define ourselves by the foods we eat, and to "lose" a food from our life is like losing a part of ourselves. We may even go through a grieving process. I think about the time I told a friend about some of the IC dietary limitations, and she said she would "die" if she couldn't have her coffee in the morning!

Similarly, since a food might bother your bladder one time but not the next, it is easy to rationalize eating the food freely again, especially if it is a food that we really miss. I did this a while back with grapefruits. When I was a child, my grandmother hooked me up with the grapefruit-a-day habit. After being diagnosed with IC, I did not eat grapefruits for a long time. Then, about 2 years ago, I bought some grapefruits for the family and tried one. It didn't bother me at all! About a week later I had another one, still without causing me problems. So, slowly the grapefruit habit snuck back into my life. Within a few months I was rushing to the doctor with what I thought was a bladder infection. You can guess by now what was happening, but it took me several weeks to concede that it was all of those grapefruits causing my IC symptoms to flare.

Redefining "Elimination Diet"

What was your reaction when you first heard the phrase "elimination diet?" Many IC patients are confused and intimidated by the thought of doing something that sounds so drastic. My first experience with an elimination diet was when my daughter, Rebekah, was two years old. Her skin was raw from eczema, so the pediatrician suggested doing an elimination diet to help determine if she had food allergies. Now, the first phase of a traditional allergy elimination diet is quite severe. She started out on lamb, pears, and rice. It was complicated to find foods a two year old would eat, while the rest of us ate "real" food. After she lost two pounds in just a few days, I stopped it.

Because of this experience, when I finally started studying the IC food lists, the idea of doing an "elimination diet" was nearly paralyzing. As a result, I did things the hard way for the next few years. I experimented with my diet, relying on trial and error, mixed with a hearty portion of denial.

It wasn't until I started counseling IC patients that I recognized the value of using an elimination diet strategy. I realized that an "elimination diet" is just a fancy way to organize the testing of various foods, and it definitely wasn't necessary to start with lamb, rice, and pears like my daughter did twenty years ago!

What follows is the system that I use with IC patients who want to sort out their trigger foods. In order to get a clear picture of which foods affect your personal IC symptoms, you need to keep good records. You might be familiar with diaries used to record your IC symptoms, and others where you record your food intake. I have included a *"Voiding and Pain Diary"* (Table 3-1) and a *"Food Intake Diary"* (Table 3-2) in this chapter. Feel free to copy them as needed or use them as a model to create charts in your personal journal. You can also download the diaries at http://www.NutraConsults.com/CCresources.html.

The IC Food List (Table 3-3) that is used was adapted from the list composed by the Interstitial Cystitis Network (http://www.ic-network.com). You will notice that the left hand column is labeled "Usually OK," the middle column is labeled "May Be OK" and the right hand column is labeled "Usually Problematic." These designations are based on years of reports from veteran IC patients and physicians. The list is not meant to be a good food/bad food list; rather it should be used as a guideline for determining your personal trigger foods. Some important things to remember when using the list:

- Most IC patients are able to eat a few of the foods listed as "problematic."
- Occasionally, patients must avoid some foods listed as "Usually OK."
- Food may have different affects on people in raw and cooked forms.
- IC patients may experience different symptoms from food at various stages of the disease.
- Pay attention to the ingredient labels of pre-packaged foods. In the beginning, avoid added preservatives, artificial sweeteners, artificial flavors and coloring.
- Avoid flavor enhancers such as monosodium glutamate (MSG).
- Read food labels. Other ingredients that signal MSG in a product are: hydrolyzed vegetable protein (HVP), hydrolyzed plant protein (HPP), natural flavoring (may have HVP), Accent, Zest, and Chinese seasoning.
- After treatment, many IC patients find that they can add back some foods in small quantities.

Preparing to Experiment

Maintaining a positive attitude during this process is extremely important. Determining your trigger foods should not be an exercise in deprivation, but rather an exercise in healing! When you take the challenge to determine your personal trigger foods, you take control of your health, and empower yourself to live as normal a life as possible.

There are three phases to this IC elimination diet strategy. Trying to figure out your trigger foods can be a mental and organizational challenge. When you have IC, you do not always have the time and energy to try new recipes and plan IC friendly meals. Because of that, I encourage you to do the first two phases of the system during a time when your calendar is relatively clear. The three phases of this process are:

- **Week One (Baseline Diet):** Record your normal food intake, pain levels, and voiding habits.
- **Weeks Two and Three (Minimal Diet):** Consume a minimal diet based on foods that are" Usually OK" for IC patients
- **Testing Period:** Test foods one at a time for three days before testing the next new food.

Week One (Baseline Diet)

It is important to know what foods you are eating and what your baseline IC symptoms are *before* you start your elimination diet. To find out your baseline, write down everything you eat, and record your IC symptoms for one week using the diaries provided. Keep good notes, especially on pain levels, food preparation methods, and other activities that may affect your IC symptoms. To standardize how you record your level of pain, you can use the *Sample Pain Scale* in Table 3-4. It isn't necessary to determine cause and effect just yet. This is just a snapshot of what is happening before you make any dietary changes.

Weeks Two and Three (Minimal Diet)

To avoid feeling deprived, it is important to eat foods that you are familiar with, especially in the beginning. Take a look at the *Sample Grocery List* (Table 3-5) that was created from the *IC Food List*. Start personalizing the grocery list by circling the foods that you like and avoiding the foods that you already suspect give you problems. You might want to make separate copies of the list for your refrigerator, for work, and to keep in your purse or wallet. Although the list may seem limited at first, in just a few weeks, you will be adding many more foods to your personal "Usually OK" list.

Over the next two weeks, only choose foods from your personalized "Usually OK" list. If you get stuck, Chapter 5 provides practical hints on meal planning. An IC Diet created from the "Usually OK" food list is not nutrient deficient if you choose food from all of the food groups. Also, please remember to keep detailed *Voiding and Pain Diaries* and *Food Intake Diaries* during this time.

Hint: To simplify recording of your food intake, use your *Food Intake Diaries* as planning sheets. Each evening, take some time to write down what you "plan" to eat the next day. Then all you have to do is record the time that you ate each meal. If you do not eat what you originally planned, just change what you wrote the night before.

Hopefully, after completing these two weeks, you will experience some relief from your IC pain and frequency. If you don't think you have reduced your symptoms significantly, compare your pain diaries from the first and fourth weeks. Again, you might not take your symptoms down to "0" or feel completely normal, but a two or three level reduction in your level of pain, and reducing the number of times you void should be considered significant improvement.

If, after you compare your diaries to previous weeks, you still do not feel you have improved significantly, you may want to consider one of these options:

- Follow the "Usually OK" diet for another week and reassess your results
- Get some help deciphering your diaries from your physician or a dietitian
- Try eating a more restrictive diet, but only under the guidance of a dietitian or your physician

Testing Period

After two weeks of limiting your food choices, you will be eager to try something new. The testing period will give you a chance to develop an expanded and personalized "Usually OK" food list.

To stay organized, I recommend that you create a list of foods that you want to try. Choose from foods that you miss the most, foods that are on the "Maybe OK" list, foods that add flavor, and foods that will improve your total nutritional intake. Examples of what you might try include:

- Blueberries
- Blackberries
- Bananas
- Onions
- Low-acid juices
- Whole wheat bread
- Almonds
- Spinach
- Yogurt
- Black Pepper

Since testing some foods might increase your symptoms temporarily, it is a good idea to choose a couple of days when you can observe your symptoms and then take it easy if your bladder flares. Usually a three-day trial is long enough to determine if a food is going to affect you or not. The rules for testing new foods are:

- Test one food at a time
- Try a small portion of the food the first day
- If you don't experience any increase in symptoms, try a larger portion the next day
- If you are still doing fine, try to eat a couple of portions of the food on the third day
- If you do not react, you can add that food to your personal "Usually Ok" food list!

If you react to a food at any time, simply record the reaction and note to try the food again later. Sometimes other things are happening in your life that can cause your bladder to flare, and when you try the food at a later date you will find that it is fine. Also, if your IC flares when trying a food, wait a day or so for your bladder symptoms to subside before trying the next food on your list. You might ask your physician about using a urinary anesthetic like Pyridium to calm your bladder if you flare from a food. Or, some patients find that dissolving a half teaspoon of baking soda in a glass of water and drinking it can temporarily quiet down their bladders, but this should not be attempted by people with sodium restriction or hypertension.

Repeating this process with each food on your list may sound like a long and tedious process, but by systematically adding foods, staying organized, and recording your symptoms, you will be more confident of your food choices.

Finally, a common question asked by patients is, "How long from mouth to bladder?" The answer is vague. It depends on the person and the food. Some foods, like cranberry juice, will likely cause a reaction within an hour. Other foods might not cause a reaction in small doses, but you could react when you increase the portion size. Some patients will experience an increase in symptoms right before bedtime and others report a day or two lag between eating a food and the development of symptoms. In most cases, however, if you are going to experience symptoms with a particular food, it will most likely happen within hours.

Taking Control

Using the IC Food List in Table 3-3, make a list of foods from each column that you like and will eat the most often.

_____
_____
_____
_____
_____
_____
_____

Using the suggestion to add back foods that you miss the most (foods that are on the "Maybe OK" list, foods that add flavor, and foods that will improve your total nutritional intake) make a list of foods that you would like to try first during the testing phase:

_____
_____
_____
_____
_____
_____
_____
_____

Staying positive and motivated is very important to the success of your elimination diet strategy. What are ways that you can stay positive and motivated? (Examples: talking with other IC patients, finding positive quotes to post around your home, at work, or in your journal; hanging a calendar with the menus planned out so you can cross off the days, or sending reminder e-mails to yourself like "keep it up!)

_____
_____
_____
_____
_____
_____
_____
_____
_____
_____
_____
_____
_____
_____

Table 3-1: Voiding and Pain Diary				
Date	Time	Volume	Pain Level (1-10)	Notes

Table 3-2 Food Intake Diary				
Date	Time	Food	Amount	Preparation

Y - Yes
N - No

Table 3-3: The IC Food List

Adapted from Interstitial Cystitis Network

Usually OK	May Be OK	Usually Problematic
Beverages		
almond milk Y chamomile tea Y Evian® water Y distilled or filtered water Y Gerber® pear juice Y milk Y mint tea Y	alfalfa tea N bottled water Y coffee substitutes Y low acid decaf coffee Y low acid juices N gin Y rice milk Y root beer w/ ice Y rum Y tap water N	beer No carbonated water N chocolate milk Y citrus juices N cranberry juice N herb teas w/rose hips most fruit juices N regular coffee Y sodas N soy milk N tea N wines N
Grains		
buckwheat corn bread Y couscous Y matzo Y millet Y oat bread Y pasta Y pitas Y potato bread Y quinoa Y rice Y spelt white bread Y	amaranth bread or cereal w/ preservatives grits Y oatmeal Y rye bread N sourdough bread Y some graham crackers w/o problem ingredients Y whole wheat bread Y	soy flour N bread or cereal with high fortification
Fats, Oils, and Nuts		
butter Y canola oil Y coconut w/o preservatives Y coconut oil Y corn oil Y margarine Y olive oil Y peanut oil sesame oil Y shortening Y soy oil N	almonds Y cashews N tahini N sunflower seeds Y	filberts hazelnuts N macadamia nuts N mayonnaise N most salad dressings peanuts N pecans Y - Little pistachio nuts N English and black walnuts N

Usually OK	May Be OK	Usually
\multicolumn{3}{c}{Soups}		
homemade soups Y from ok meats and vegetables	Health Valley® chicken broth some canned soups w/o problem ingredients	bouillon cubes N bouillon powder most packaged and N canned soups
\multicolumn{3}{c}{Meats, Fish, Poultry, and Protein}		
beef Y chicken Y dried beans, peas, lentils Y eggs Y fish Y ~~lamb~~ liver (beef or chicken) Y pork Y shellfish Y shrimp Y turkey Y veal Y	anchovies N bacon Y Canadian bacon Y ~~caviar~~ corned beef N liverwurst Y some sausages Y w/o problem ingredients	bologna N ham N hot dogs N most sausage N pepperoni N salami N smoked fish N
\multicolumn{3}{c}{Dairy}		
cream cheese Y cottage cheese Y feta Y mozzarella Y ricotta Y string cheeses Y whipped cream Y vanilla ice cream Y	buttermilk Y parmesan Y Cool Whip® Y Monterey jack Y some sherbets N some frozen yogurt Y Rice Dream® Y	aged cheeses N blue cheese N brie N brick parmesan Y camembert N cheddar Y edam N gruyer N montery jack Y roquefort N sorbet N soy milk N soy cheese N sour cream N stilton N swiss N yogurt yes

Usually OK	May Be OK	Usually Problem
Vegetables		
broccoli Y brussel sprouts Y cabbage Y carrots Y cauliflower Y celery Y chives Y collard greens N corn Y cucumber Y green beans Y kale Y lettuce Y mushrooms Y okra Y parsley Y peas Y potatoes Y pumpkin Y radishes Y snow peas Y split peas Y summer squash Y turnips Y winter squash Y yams Y yellow beans Y zucchini Y	avocado Y beets Y chicory cooked bulb onions Y cooked leeks N dandelion greens eggplant Y low-acid tomatoes N raw green onions Tops rhubarb N rutabagas Y swiss chard N spinach Y turnip greens N	chili peppers N fava beans N lima beans N pickles N raw bulb onions N sauerkraut N soy beans) N tomato N tomato sauces N
Fruits		
dates w/o preservatives Y coconut w/o preservatives Y pears Y	bananas Y blueberries Y ~~brown raisins~~ cherimoya citrus peels H crenshaw melon ~~dried currants~~ Gala apples Y honeydew Y mango (small amt) N maraschino cherries Y rhubarb N watermelon Y	apricots N all citrus fruit N cantaloupe N cherries N peaches N most plums N most dried figs N golden raisins N grapes N guava N kiwi fruit N most berries N passion fruit N papaya N persimmon N pineapple N star fruit N

Usually OK	May Be OK	Usually Problematic
Sweets and Desserts		
brown sugar y carob carrot cake y crème brule y custards y divinity homemade pound cake y homemade white and yellow cakes y homemade vanilla frosting y homemade caramel frosting y honey y licorice y maple syrup y pear pastries y sugar y sugar cookies y tapioca y vanilla ice cream y vanilla pudding y	banana bread y blueberry pastries y caramel candies y peppermint ice cream y plain pastries w/ almonds y plain cheesecakes y some frozen yogurt y some hard candies w/o acids y some popsicles Splenda® N (sucralose) stevia y white chocolate y	acesulfame K N aspartame N catsup N chocolate y coffee ice cream N desserts w/ problem nuts N pastries w/ problem fruits N pecan pie N sorbets N store-bought fruitcakes N mincemeat pie N Nutrasweet® N saccharine N
Seasonings and Additives		
allspice y almond extract y anise y basil y caraway seed y coriander y dill y fennel y garlic y mace y marjoram N oregano y poppy seed N rosemary y sage y salt y thyme y tarragon y vanilla extract y	black pepper y celery seed y cilantro y cinnamon y cumin (small amt) N dried parsley y dried chervil N ginger ? N lemon extract N malt powder nutmeg y onion powder y orange extract y turmeric N	ascorbic acid N autolyzed yeast N BHA and BHT N benzoates N caffeine N cayenne N chili powder N citric acid N cloves N hot curry powder N hydrolyzed protein N meat tenderizers N metabisulfites N MSG (monosodium glutamate) N mustard N oleoresin paprika N paprika N red pepper N soy sauce N sulfites N tamari N vinegar N Worcestershire sauce N

Table 3-4: Sample Pain Scale

Level 1: I feel no symptoms of IC. I can do anything.

Level 2: I feel slight discomfort, possibly the beginning of a flare. I can do anything.

Level 3: I feel mild symptoms of IC. It is not stopping me from my daily life but I am feeling some mild discomfort.

Level 4: I feel moderate symptoms of IC and have a moderate need to urinate, with a moderate level of pain. My activities are limited. My frequency is higher, and I am looking for restrooms and using them. At this point, I am on my way home to rest and begin my pain management strategies and/or medication.

Level 5: I am very uncomfortable, perhaps biting my lip and/or holding my abdomen. I am usually laying in bed now. Walking is more painful now. IC has limited me from doing my daily functions. I am utilizing some of my pain management medications and tools at this point.

Level 6: I am having constant intense pelvic pain with moderate frequency and urgency. I am worried and ready to call my doctor for advice.

Level 7: I am in bed in severe pain. I am using all of my coping strategies, but I may need help at this point. I am considering calling my doctor and may go to the emergency room for help.

Level 8: I am having difficulty tolerating the pain. I am calling my doctor.

Level 9: Pain is intolerable; I am on my way to the emergency room because I need help in managing my pain.

Level 10: Excruciating pain

Reprinted with permission from Interstitial Cystitis Network

Table 3-5 Sample Grocery List	
Fresh Fruits	
Pears	Blueberries
Coconut (no preservatives)	Dates (no preservatives)
Fresh Vegetables	
Broccoli	Brussel sprouts
Fresh oregano	Cabbage
Fresh garlic	Carrots
Fresh basil	Baby carrots
Zucchini	Cauliflower
Yams	Chives
Sweet Potatoes	Greens
Turnips	Corn
Cucumber	Mushrooms
Okra	Lettuce and other salad greens
Parsley	Peas
Pumpkin	Squash
Radishes	Potatoes
	Snow peas

Canned Fruits/Juices	
Canned Pears	Gerber pear juice
Organic blueberry juice	Gerber baby food pears

Canned Vegetables	
Carrots	Corn
Kidney beans	Greens
Black beans	Green or yellow beans
Navy beans	Mushrooms
Peas	Yams
Sweet potatoes	Pumpkin

Frozen Goods	
Broccoli	Carrots
Vanilla ice cream	Corn
Blueberries	Peas
	Mixed vegetables

Oils, Fats, and Nuts	
Olive oil	Canola or other vegetable oil
Butter	Shortening (trans-fat free)
Margarine	Cooking spray

Dairy and Eggs

Milk (preferably non-fat)	Evaporated skim milk
Cream cheese	Dried milk
String cheese	Feta cheese
Ricotta	Mozzarella cheese
	Whipped cream

Baking Products

Flour	Sugar
Almond extract	Honey
Natural vanilla extract	Corn meal
Maple syrup	Muffin mix
Vanilla frosting	Baking soda
Vanilla pudding	Baking powder
Caramel	Carob powder
White chocolate chips	Carob chips

Seasonings

Allspice	Anise
Caraway seed	Basil
Tarragon	Poppy Seed
Rosemary	Marjoram
Sage	Dill
Salt	Fennel
Thyme	Garlic salt or powder
Oregano	Mace

Dried Goods	
Long grain rice	Instant rice
Elbow macaroni	Mashed potato flakes
Linguini	Dried beans, lentils, or peas
Angel hair pasta	Egg noodles
Pasta shells	Spaghetti

Breads/Snacks	
White bread	Oat bread
Vanilla wafers	Pita bread
All natural potato chips	English muffins
All natural pretzels	Bagels
Sugar candy in "safe" flavors	Blueberry muffins
Marshmallows	Sugar cookies
	Carob malt balls

Meats	
Shrimp	Chicken
Lobster	Fish
Scallops	Lamb
Turkey	Liver
Veal	Pork
	Crab

Miscellaneous	
Paper plates	Paper napkins
Paper bowls	Disposable utensils
Paper Towels	Zipper bags for freezing

5

Planning Meals

*"You don't have to cook fancy or complicated masterpieces –
just good food from fresh ingredients."*
Julia Child

A Road Map

Imagine that you are going to take a vacation. If you are like most people, you probably start choosing a destination weeks or even months in advance. You will likely spend time deciding on transportation, entertainment, and lodging. If you are driving, you might study road maps to familiarize yourself with the various routes you can take; or if you are flying, you might compare the price and convenience of various airlines.

Now imagine the confusion and frustration that would result if you just woke up one day and decided to take a vacation. Just choosing where you want to go would be paralyzing, let alone knowing what to pack for clothes, or arranging last minute transportation. Of course, you can drive to your destination, but will you get there without a map or directions?

Just like planning a vacation, spending a few minutes each week planning IC friendly meals can save you the agony of making last minute decisions. Having meals planned in advance can even reduce the temptation to eat outside of the home. Also, creating a grocery list from your menus and shopping once a week, will save you the frustration of shuffling the contents of your refrigerator and pantry or running to the store at the last minute to find that one elusive ingredient.

Good Nutrition with IC

There certainly are concerns about consuming healthy foods anytime your diet is restricted. Some people even turn to comfort foods when they are ill, rationalizing that they are sick anyway, why does it matter what they eat? Many others, however, find that having to modify their diet for a particular health condition causes them to consider eating better than they had before their illness.

One of the biggest concerns expressed by IC patients when they first look at any version of the IC diet is that the fruit selections appear to be very slim. It certainly seems odd that one of the healthiest foods for most people is "forbidden" for people who are trying to get well.

That concern is valid. Fruits and vegetables are as close to a magic bullet that we have when it comes to preventing heart disease, cancer, diabetes, stroke, obesity, and even various forms of dementia like Alzheimer's. We are not just talking about the vitamins in fruit and vegetables either. In the past 20 years, nutrition science has discovered some exciting substances in plant foods that they call phytochemicals. These substances act as antioxidants in our bodies, protecting the cells from damage of free radicals. Simply put, phytochemicals in fruits and vegetables clean up the garbage in our bodies that can cause many diseases.

So what is an IC patient to do? Well, the first thing to remember is that most IC patients can eat more than the traditional pears and blueberries. Many people report being able to eat raspberries, bananas, apples, and even some grapes occasionally. The key is for you to try one fruit at a time when you are feeling good enough to tell the difference if you flare. Also, remember that many flares from food are dose related. In other words, a half of an apple twice a week is less likely to bother you than an apple a day. Similarly, a small squeeze of lemon in a glass of water may not cause you the same misery as a glass of lemonade. Of course, using an antacid product like Prelief or pH Control (refer to Chapter 15) may allow you to eat a larger variety of fruits.

If you find you are legitimately sensitive to most fruits, it is good to know that many vegetables provide the same or similar phytochemicals and vitamins. Phytochemicals form the color pigments of plants, so chose brightly colored vegetables like carrots, broccoli, red cabbage, spinach, squash, pumpkin, yams, and sweet potatoes. Although it may be tempting to take a vitamin or supplement, scientists estimate that there are 100,000 different phytochemicals and, to date, we only know the properties of about 200 of them! If we only take "pills" filled with the ones we know about, what amazing things are we throwing away? There is also ample evidence that taking megadoses of some phytochemicals can actually cause cellular damage. So, to be safe, it is best to get your daily dose of nutrients from food.

On that note, I have included this *Food Groups for Healthy Eating* to guide your food choices:

Food Groups for Healthy Eating

Food Group	# Per Day	Serving Sizes
Dairy	2-3	1 c. low-fat milk 1 c. yogurt (if tolerated) 1 ½ oz. low-fat soft cheese
Fruits	3-4	1 medium pear 2 canned pear halves 3/4 c. blueberries 1/4 c. dried dates without preservatives 1/2 c. frozen blueberries
Vegetables	3-5	1/2 c. cooked 1 c. raw, or salad
Grains	5-8	1 slice bread 1/2 c. dry or hot cereal 1/2 c. cooked rice or pasta
Meats/Protein	3 or less	3 oz. cooked meat, poultry, fish 1-2 eggs 1/2 c. legumes
Nuts/Seeds	4 per week	1/3 c. nuts 2 T. seeds
Sweets/fats	limited	olive oil peanut oil canola oil sugar, brown sugar honey maple syrup

Keeping it Simple

If you are just beginning to use an elimination diet to determine your food triggers, you can design menus using your "Usually OK" food list. It is also important to keep your meals as plain and simple as possible. It is much harder to filter out which food is causing your symptoms to flare if you are eating foods with many ingredients such as casseroles, soups, or stir-fries. Other hints for keeping it simple at this stage include:

- Make menu planning a family affair. Consulting with other family members about menu choices can increase their understanding of your condition.

- Consider including foods that might be triggers for you, but that your family can eat. It was nearly a year before I realized that I had not been buying strawberries for my family just because I couldn't have them!

- Stick to your grocery list. Often people walk through the grocery store waiting for inspiration to strike. A list insures that you have all the ingredients that you need for the week and helps prevent impulse buying, which can be tough on the wallet.

- Recycle your weekly meal plans like institutions do. Hospitals, schools, and nursing homes use "cycle menus" to simplify planning. Once you have developed a few weeks of menus that you and your family enjoy, go ahead and reuse them. Save the grocery lists, too!

- Do your grocery shopping from your computer. Companies like "WeGoShop.com" allow you to send a grocery order to a professional shopper who brings your order directly to your house (www.wegoshop.com). This can be a great time and energy saver.

- Make two batches of a meal and freeze one for later. Everyone has days when they are too busy or too tired to cook. It is nice to have something available that you can quickly reheat.

- Involve everyone in mealtime activities. Establish this as a special time to spend with individual family members. Assign days when each person has a chance to help with breakfast or dinner. Have all the ingredients out for people to pack their own lunches. Even small children can help to set the table, measure ingredients or stir batter.

- Simplify cleanup. Use disposable plates and utensils on days when symptoms flare or energy is limited. Line baking dishes with aluminum foil or bake food in foil pockets. Use a slow cooker to bake a one pot, complete meal of meat, potatoes, and vegetables.

Some Notes on Eating Out

Having a chronic illness can deplete your time and energy, and it can be tempting to order in or eat out. However, eating meals away from home is not always a time saver. Waiting in line for fast food or sitting down to eat at a restaurant often takes just as long as preparing a simple meal at home. It is also much easier to control the ingredients and seasonings in foods that you prepare yourself.

Of course, there will be times when you need to eat outside of the home. Even if your diet is limited, there are steps you can take to make sure the food you eat is as safe for you as possible. Fast food restaurants offer plain hamburgers and milk or milk shakes in a pinch. Most other restaurants will gladly accommodate special orders from their customers. At the very least you should be able to order plain baked chicken, baked potato or white rice, and vegetables.

Navigating food choices in other people's homes, on holidays, or at events like weddings can be slightly more difficult. Your best strategy is to find out ahead of time what is being served and work around it. If you know in advance that the food choices will not be IC friendly, eat a sandwich or small meal before you go. You can also offer to take a dish to pass, if that is appropriate for the situation.

Snack Tips

Snacking has become a way of life for most people, and snack food advertising alone is a multi-billion dollar industry. Certainly, many snack options are high fat and high sugar, but carefully chosen snacks can be an important part of a daily meal plan. Here are a few hints to help you choose wisely:

- Plan your snacks ahead of time like you do your meals.
- Choose high nutrient foods such as celery, carrots, cauliflower, broccoli, cucumbers, blueberries, and pears.
- Try homemade vegetable muffins, such as pumpkin, carrot, or zucchini.
- Keep IC friendly pretzels, vanilla wafers, animal crackers, cereals, corn or rice cakes, and popcorn on hand for quick, crunchy snacks.
- Reach for a protein snack such as cottage cheese, string cheese, hard-boiled eggs, or even a sandwich if a meal is delayed.
- Make homemade milk shakes in your blender with low-fat vanilla ice cream, skim milk, ice cubes, and a touch of natural almond or vanilla extract.
- Other snack options include caramels, carob malt balls or coated raisins, and homemade white chocolate chip cookies.

You Can Plan

Planning your meals ahead of time and making a weekly grocery list based on that plan can help you eat healthier, keep you on track with IC friendly foods, and reduce mealtime frustration. Taking the time to plan meals can also increase satisfaction with your meals, despite the dietary limitations of an IC diet.

Taking Control

What is your current meal schedule?

_____
_____
_____
_____

How many meals do you consume from home each week? Include meals prepared at home but eaten away.

_____
_____
_____
_____

How many meals do you eat from outside sources?

_____
_____
_____
_____

If you eat meals outside the home, where are you eating? What are you eating?

_____
_____
_____
_____
_____

What foods can you keep on hand for snacks?

_____
_____
_____
_____
_____

How can other family members participate in meal preparation? How can everyone make this a pleasant time?

_____
_____
_____
_____
_____

6

Breakfast

"'When you wake up in the morning, Pooh,' said Piglet at last, 'what's the first thing you say to yourself?' 'What's for breakfast?' said Pooh. 'What do you say, Piglet?' 'I say, I wonder what's going to happen exciting today?' said Piglet. Pooh nodded thoughtfully. 'It's the same thing,' he said."
A. A. Milne, *The House at Pooh Corner*

Why Breakfast?

Although most of us know better, up to a third of US adults still report skipping breakfast on any given day. So why is breakfast so important? Well, the simple explanation is that after "fasting" through the night, breakfast provides you with the fuel to begin your day. People who eat breakfast generally burn more calories, and consume more fiber, calcium, and iron than those who skip breakfast. In addition, those who have breakfast eat fewer calories per day than breakfast skippers. In general, breakfast eaters also have lower cholesterol levels.

However, the effects of eating breakfast are more than physical. Eating breakfast contributes to increased alertness, higher scores on short-term memory tests, and sharper problem solving skills. People who eat breakfast also report lower stress levels and less depression than those who miss breakfast. As a rule, eating breakfast can increase the quality of your daily performance.

The good news for IC patients is that breakfast is often the easiest meal to manage. Although some foods are restricted in the first few weeks of the elimination diet, eventually, many people find they can reintroduce typical breakfast foods including certain fruits, low-acid juices, and oatmeal. Some patients may even be able to drink low-acid, decaffeinated coffee occasionally.

There are some specific breakfast foods that you should watch out for. Sausages and other breakfast-type meats usually have high levels of nitrates and other preservatives. You may find some organic sausages or bacons will work for you. Also, some cereals are highly fortified with vitamins. Since many IC patients are extremely sensitive to "mega" doses of vitamins, you should avoid cereals that claim to have 100% of any nutrient, especially vitamin C and the B vitamins.

What if you are not hungry in the morning or you feel you do not have time to prepare a meal? Instead of grabbing a doughnut, which will only leave you hungrier in the long run, try having a glass of milk or a slice of toast first thing in the morning. Then, in an hour or so, have a hard-boiled egg or a half-cup of cottage cheese. If you do not like traditional breakfast foods, go ahead and eat a turkey sandwich, a slice of mozzarella melted over half a bagel, or even a cup of chicken and rice soup!

Sample Breakfast Menus

You will find many breakfast ideas in your favorite cookbooks. Since you control the ingredients, homemade breakfast foods can be more nutritious and IC friendly than foods purchased in a store. Eight sample breakfast menus are included here to get you started:

Breakfast 1
   1 or 2 eggs, any style
   2 slices of (white bread) toast
   Butter, margarine, or blueberry jam
   6 oz. of pear juice

Breakfast 2
   2 slices of french toast
   Maple syrup
   ½ c. cottage cheese
   6 oz. organic blueberry juice

Breakfast 3
   ¾ c. cold or hot cereal (no preservatives)
   ½ c. low-fat milk
   ¼ c. fresh blueberries, sweetened with sugar as desired

Breakfast 4
   1 or 2 eggs, any style
   ¾ c. home fried potatoes (seasoned with salt)
   1 oz. corn bread
   ¾ c. pears

Breakfast 5
   Homemade blueberry pancakes (page 97)
   Blueberry syrup
   1 T. butter, margarine, or fresh, sweetened whipped cream
   6 oz. pear juice

Breakfast 6
   2 egg omelet (eggs, feta cheese, mushrooms, chopped broccoli or other vegetable)
   2 slices of toast (white bread) with butter, margarine, or Blueberry "Jam" (page 86)
   6 oz. organic blueberry juice

Breakfast 7

Homemade waffles
Pear sauce (Heat in sauce pan over medium heat until the fruit is a chunky consistency similar to applesauce: 2 sliced pears, ¼ c. sugar, 1 T. brown sugar, and 1 T. water)
1 T. butter
1 c. low-fat milk

Breakfast 8

Breakfast stuffed pita
  ½ pita bread
  1 scrambled egg
  1 T. feta cheese
  ¼ c. sliced sautéed mushrooms
1 c. fresh pear slices
1 c. low-fat milk

Taking Control

What can you do to start creating breakfasts that would be a healthy addition to your lifestyle?

_____
_____
_____
_____
_____
_____
_____
_____
_____
_____
_____

Plan a week's worth of breakfasts using your personal IC "Usually OK" food list:

What groceries do you need to have on hand for the breakfasts that you planned?

Using your food diary or journal, record your experiences following your breakfast meal plans. If you change your original plan, or if you eat something that was not planned, be sure to record what you actually ate.

7

Lunch

"Too few people understand a really good sandwich."
James Beard

Making Time for Lunch

Naturally, good eating habits should not stop with breakfast. Eating regular meals throughout the day is vital for sustaining physical energy, supporting mental acuity, and managing weight. Poor eating habits can contribute to heart disease, obesity, osteoporosis, and diabetes, yet too many people find it easy to skip lunch. Others sacrifice nutritional needs, choosing junk food or high fat and high calorie fast foods.

Yet, a healthy, IC friendly lunch does not have to take hours to prepare or be boring to eat. By including lunches in your weekly meal plan and grocery list, you can alleviate the frustration and confusion of making lunchtime food choices at the last minute. Also, consider packaging individual portions of vegetables, sandwich meats, bread and snacks a week in advance so it's not a chore to do each day. Just grab what you need each day and go.

To avoid adding to the morning chaos, pack brown-bag lunches the night before. You can even wait to assemble your sandwich right before you eat. If you have a refrigerator and microwave available at lunch, pack soup or leftovers as you are cleaning up after dinner. Purchase individual containers of milk from employee cafeterias or even drive through restaurants (if you can avoid the temptation to buy anything else!)

Making Lunch Exciting (and Healthy)

No one wants to eat a turkey sandwich and carrot sticks everyday. Get creative as you plan your meals each week. Make a list of foods from the various food groups that you can combine in various ways. For example, a simple way to reduce the monotony of cold sandwiches is to experiment with different breads. Selecting foods from all of the food groups is also an excellent way to be sure that you are getting all the nutrients you need. Here are some suggestions from each group:

Milk and Dairy Products
- Low-fat or fat-free milk
- Cottage cheese
- String cheese
- Mozzarella cheese slices
- Feta cheese for pocket sandwiches or salads

Fruit and Vegetables
- Cut vegetables: carrots, celery, broccoli, cucumber, etc.
- Sandwich fillers: mushrooms, parsley, lettuce, lentils, corn, chives, carrots, etc.
- Salad toppings: carrots, broccoli, mushrooms, chives
- Fresh pears and blueberries
- Dates (without preservatives)
- Pear and blueberry cobblers or pastries

Breads and Starches
- Pita bread
- Hot dog or hamburger rolls
- Corn bread muffins
- Blueberry muffins
- Carrot or zucchini muffins or breads (shredded vegetables added to basic muffin recipe)
- Pasta
- Oat bread
- White bread

Meat and Other Protein Foods
- Homemade meat and vegetable soups
- Fresh cooked chicken, beef, cold shrimp, or turkey for salads or sandwiches (no processed meats)
- Hard boiled eggs, sliced and chopped for salads or sandwiches
- Red beans, navy beans, black beans for salads, side dishes, or sandwich fillings

Condiments and Flavorings
- Fresh basil, tarragon, garlic, sage, or rosemary
- Salt, sugar, pepper (if tolerated)
- Butter or margarine
- Olive oil, peanut oil, canola oil
- MSG free broths
- Homemade salad dressings (try replacing pear juice for vinegar in recipes)

Beverages
- Ice water
- Milk
- Almond milk
- Mint or chamomile tea (hot or iced)
- Pear juice

Sample Lunch Menus

Planning and preparing your lunches in advance can help reduce any temptation you might have to grab fast food or raid vending machines, habits which can compromise your health and interfere with your attempts to sort out your personal trigger foods. Sample lunch menus are included here to get you started:

Lunch 1

    Chicken Wrap Sandwich
        flat bread wrap
        chopped chicken
        bean sprouts, shredded carrots, cucumber
Pear
1 c. low-fat milk
Sugar cookie

Lunch 2

    Homemade beef and vegetable soup
    Cornbread muffin
    ¾ c. blueberries (fresh or frozen)
    1 c. low-fat milk

Lunch 3

    Turkey and feta salad
        Lettuce and other greens
        Turkey
        Feta cheese
        Chopped hard boiled egg
        Salad dressing made from olive oil, pear juice, sugar, basil, salt
White bread dinner roll with butter or honey
1 c. low-fat milk
¾ c. vanilla ice cream

Lunch 4

    Pasta Salad
        Cooked chilled pasta
        Broccoli
        Shredded mozzarella cheese
        Shredded carrots
        Cooked, chopped chicken
    1 slice bread with butter, margarine, or blueberry jam
    1 c. low-fat milk
    1 small piece yellow cake with vanilla frosting

Lunch 5

    Turkey sandwich (lettuce, butter)
    Pear
    Carrot and celery sticks
    Tapioca pudding
    1 c. low-fat milk

Lunch 6

    Tuna steak on a bun (broiled, salt ok)
    Oven fries
    ¾ c. green beans
    1 c. low-fat milk
    Carrot cake

Lunch 7

    Homemade chicken and rice soup
    Blueberry Muffin (page 103)
    1 c. low-fat milk
    Carob chip cookie

Lunch 8
    Roast beef and mozzarella melt
        1/2 bagel
        2 oz. of sliced roast beef
        1 oz. slice mozzarella
        (Layer and broil until cheese is bubbly
    Peas and carrots
    Butterscotch Brownie (page 94)

Taking Control

What type of foods do you usually eat for lunch?

_____
_____
_____
_____
_____
_____

Where do you usually eat your lunch? What preparation facilities do you have available? (Example: refrigerator, freezer, microwave, or stovetop)

_____
_____
_____
_____
_____
_____
_____
_____

Plan a week's worth of lunches using your personal IC "OK" food list. Consider your schedule and the tasks necessary to prepare your meals:

___

What groceries do you need to have on hand for the lunches that you planned?

___

Using your food diary or journal, record your experiences following your lunch meal plans. If you change your original plan, or if you eat something that was not planned, be sure to record what you actually ate:

___

8

Dinner

"Strange to see how a good dinner and feasting reconciles everybody."
Samuel Pepys

The Balancing Act

For many people, evening is a busy but pleasant time when they catch up on chores, take part in sports or hobbies, cook, and share a meal with their family. If you have IC, however, sometimes the tasks at the end of the day can be overwhelming. Fortunately, with a little bit of planning, balancing your evening activities does not mean you will have to give up home cooked meals.

The first thing to remember is to take advantage of the days when you are feeling your best. Prepare double batches (or more) of a meal and freeze the extra to use on days when you are too busy or tired to cook. Similarly, some people save time and energy by preparing two, three, or even four weeks of meals on one day.

Remember, simplicity is the rule. Choose entrees with fewer than six ingredients. Experiment with a slow cooker. Beef, chicken, and even turkey breasts can be simmered all day with potatoes and vegetables, gradually filling the house with a mouth-watering aroma.

If you are the primary cook, take it easy on yourself. Peeling and cutting vegetables can be done sitting at the kitchen table. Consider using pre-cut ingredients, or purchase salads from restaurants to take home to add to your meal. Finally, many common breakfast foods like eggs or French toast are quick and nutritious, and can be a comforting meal to share with your family at the end the day.

Sample Dinner Menus

Nine sample dinner menus are included here to get you started: Remember to keep it simple, and have fun as you wind down at the end of the day.

Dinner 1
Pear Smothered Pork Chops (page 87)
Peas and mushrooms
Baked potato (butter, salt, basil)
1 c. low-fat milk
¾ c. blueberries

Dinner 2
Italian Baked Chicken (page 88)
Bow tie pasta with butter or margarine
Broccoli
1 c. low-fat milk
Vanilla pudding

Dinner 3
> Linguine with Clam Sauce (page 89)
> Sautéed zucchini and summer squash
> Dinner salad:
> > Lettuce
> > Shredded carrots
> > Cucumber slices
> > Shredded mozzarella
> > Flavored olive oil
>
> 1 c. low-fat milk
> Divinity fudge

Dinner 4
> Baked or broiled white fish
> Boiled red skin potatoes with olive oil, salt and rosemary
> Carrot Salad with Honey Dressing (page 88)
> 1 c. low-fat milk
> Scottish Shortbread (page 91)

Dinner 5
> Honey Sesame Chicken (page 91)
> White rice
> Broccoli with Garlic and Mushrooms (page 99)
> 1 c. low-fat milk
> Fortune cookies

Dinner 6
> Rosemary Beef (page 98)
> Long Grain Rice with Peas (page 99)
> Salad with dressing
> 1 c. low-fat milk
> Canned pear slices

Dinner 7
- Baked chicken
- Mashed potatoes
- Homemade gravy
- Winter squash
- 1 c. low-fat milk
- Crunchy Cookie (page 93)

Dinner 8
- Shrimp, stir fried in olive oil, garlic, seasoned with salt
- White rice
- Green beans
- Homemade biscuits and honey
- 1 c. low-fat milk

Dinner 9
- Quick White Pizza (page 105)
- Salad
- Homemade garlic bread
- 1 c. low-fat milk
- Blueberry & Pear Cobbler (page 96)

Taking Control

What type of foods do you usually eat for dinner?

_____
_____
_____
_____
_____
_____
_____
_____
_____

Plan a week's worth of dinners using your personal IC "Usually OK" food list:

_____
_____
_____
_____
_____
_____
_____
_____

What groceries do you need to have on hand to prepare the dinners you planned?

_____
_____
_____
_____
_____
_____
_____
_____

Using your food diary or journal, record your experiences following your dinner plans. If you change your original plan, or if you eat something that was not planned, be sure to record what you actually ate:

_____
_____
_____
_____
_____

9

Beverages

"Water, taken in moderation, cannot hurt anybody."
Mark Twain

What Can I Drink?

Almost certainly, the number one dietary frustration among IC patients is the scarcity of "safe" beverages, especially when they are first beginning to decipher their personal trigger foods. A quick glance at the *IC Food List* shows that the "Usually OK" list of beverages is, indeed, quite limited: chamomile tea, Evian water, distilled water, Gerber pear juice, milk, and mint tea.

Then there is the "Usually Problematic" or "forbidden" beverage category: coffee, tea, sodas, juices, and alcoholic beverages. It is easy to see why people go through denial about how beverages affect their IC symptoms; it appears that all the "fun" stuff has been taken away!

This is why you should try adding a few other beverages early in the testing phase. In all likelihood, there will be several other beverages that you can consume regularly, and even more in smaller quantities or with slight modifications. So, just as you have done with the foods, make a list of the beverages that you miss the most and make a plan to test them to see if there is an effect on your bladder. Please use the suggestions here only as a guide, remembering that most of the information on beverages and IC was collected from other patients. As with anything else, your reaction to specific foods and beverages is highly individualized and may even change over time.

Drink Right to Feel Right

Most health professionals suggest that a person needs 64 ounces of liquid a day. Maintaining proper hydration is essential for every part of the body to function properly. Our lungs, heart, brain, and even our joints are all dependent on how much fluid we drink. Although most people do get plenty to drink these days, IC patients are frequently tempted to reduce their fluid intake, believing that they will reduce the time spent in the bathroom. At first glance, this may appear to make sense, but it can be dangerous to dehydrate yourself just to avoid the bathroom. The fact is that IC patients who do this are actually concentrating their urine, potentially creating more pain for themselves in the long run. So, what should an IC patient drink?

Water

Water may seem like a simple beverage, but it is surprising how different varieties affect different people. Most people do very well with distilled or filtered tap water. If you choose to drink bottled water, be sure that it is 100% pure spring water without added minerals. Many IC patients find it easier to sip a glass of water over an hour rather than drink it all at one time. Also, try hot water with a bit of honey.

Milk

Dairy beverages are usually well tolerated by IC patients. This includes milk, low fat milk, and homemade vanilla milk shakes (For a milk shake just put ½ c. vanilla ice cream, ½ c. skim milk, 4-5 ice cubes, and a dash of vanilla extract into a blender and buzz it. Within minutes you have a wonderful treat!). Many IC patients also report good luck drinking almond milk, which is available in many grocery stores.

If you find that you can tolerate some fruits, like blueberries or raspberries, try adding them to your milk shakes in order to enhance your intake of nutrients. In addition, if you find that yogurt is not a trigger food for you, you can try yogurt smoothies. Just substitute yogurt for the ice cream in the shake recipe. Those who would like to add protein to their shakes or smoothies should avoid soy powders and opt for 100% pure whey powder since soy is often a trigger food for IC patients. Finally, people who are allergic to dairy or lactose intolerant might want to avoid soymilk and try rice milk instead.

Fruit Juice

It seems like every IC patient has a cranberry juice story. Before I was diagnosed, and I thought I was dealing with impossibly resistant urinary tract infections, I drank gallons of cranberry juice, believing it would help fight the "infections." I even resorted to cranberry extract pills from the health food store to avoid consuming all the sugar and calories of the cranberry juice. There are also plenty of IC patients whose well-meaning friends or relatives insist that the cranberry juice would cure their IC. Sometimes it is worth explaining; sometimes it isn't.

It isn't just cranberry juice, however, that can cause trouble for an IC bladder. Most people will react the same with other juices, at least until they get their symptoms under control. Pear juice is the exception since it seems to create the least problems. Organic blueberry juice is also well tolerated by many people. As you begin to test other foods, you may even find that you can add low-acid orange juice, or consume various juices in small quantities.

> *"In my experience as a support group leader, the great majority of patients who contact our office, crying in pain, usually admit to drinking coffee, soda, or green tea each day. Our best suggestion? Stop all coffees, teas, and sodas for at least a month!"*
> Jill Osborn, President
> Interstitial Cystitis Network

Coffee

Coffee and the cultural rituals associated with it are genuinely very hard to give up. People start their day with coffee, take coffee breaks at work, and socialize over coffee and dessert. In fact, I have heard IC patients say that they will do everything I tell them, but they will not give up their coffee. Of course, those who are successful in eliminating coffee from their diet usually experience significant relief.

There is good news, however. Once you have your IC symptoms under control, you may want to try coffee again, albeit slightly modified. There are several things you can do to minimize any problems you might have. One is to experiment with reduced acid, decaffeinated coffees such as Puroast (http://www.puroast.com). The producers of low acid coffees use different processing methods than other coffee producers. Other people have luck with diluting decaffeinated coffee with hot water and adding milk to balance the acid. Still others enjoy coffee substitutes such as Pero, Teeccino, and Cafix. Other possible options are to try espresso or use a "toddy" maker (available at http://www.icnshop.com) which produces a coffee with 2/3 less acid than hot brewed coffee. Rachel, a nurse and IC patient explains it this way:

> "Coffee depends on where I get it. I can't drink coffee from the local mini-marts, but, I can drink a latte from a local coffee shop. Yes, it's more expensive, but the acidity depends on the amount of time the beans are in contact with the water. The drip at the mini-mart sits there all day. To make espresso, the water is pulled through the grinds, so I can tolerate that and not have to give up my coffee! Of course, if my bladder is already flaring, I don't consume any type of coffee until my IC symptoms are in control again."

Tea

Despite the news that teas can be healthy for you, most IC patients consider tea, especially green tea, to be hazardous to their bladders. Many herbal teas are also suspect, with the exception of chamomile and mint teas. Herbal blends often contain irritating ingredients like rose hips and hibiscus leaves. You may want to try some blueberry or raspberry teas, but as with any food or beverage, pay attention to your symptoms.

Carbonated Beverages

It doesn't matter if you call these beverages pop, soda, or something else, carbonated beverages can be intense bladder irritants. Like coffee, these beverages are very hard to sacrifice, but eliminating them from your diet can be extremely beneficial. In most cases, the culprit ingredients are caffeine, citric acid, preservatives, and artificial sweeteners. Since most carbonated beverages do not have any real nutritional value, these are some of the last beverages you should attempt to add back to your diet.

Alcoholic Beverages

This is another category of beverages that just is not worth trying unless your symptoms are under control. Even though some hard liquor is on the "May Be OK" list, most IC patients find that even a small amount of alcohol can cause a flare in symptoms. Of course, people ask, "What do I drink when I celebrate or go out with friends?" I believe a good analogy comes from what we tell our youth about drinking. When you socialize, don't feel that you need to drink just to fit in. After all, if your friends understand how drinking alcohol affects you, they certainly would not want to ruin your evening.

Just in case someone raises a question regarding your choice of beverage, and you don't feel comfortable discussing the details of IC, feel free to use any of the following "excuses":

- "I might have something later; right now I am just very thirsty."
- "I am on some medications right now that can interact with alcohol."
- "I nominated myself to be the designated driver."

Or, as a response to a really insistent pal:

- "It seems that what I am drinking is more important to you than it is to me!" Then smile confidently and change the subject!

Have Patience

About a year ago I had dinner with two other IC patients. We talked about whether sodas actually bothered our bladders, and for the most part, we felt (through experience) if we take care of our bladders in other ways, a soda every two weeks or so isn't going to put us over the edge. When we sense that our IC symptoms were getting out of control, we eliminate the offending foods and drinks again.

The point is, until we get more research on diet and IC, we are limited to what we can find out ourselves. Now, I am not telling you to run out and buy a twelve pack of diet cola. In fact my message is just the opposite. First you must take the time to sort out which beverages cause you trouble. Then you might be able to increase your tolerance for some coffees, low-acid juices, and even small amounts of carbonated beverages. If you find yourself actively symptomatic, eliminate the offending beverage and drink water for a while.

Taking Control:

What beverages do you feel affect your bladder symptoms?

Make a list of beverages that you would like, but are afraid to drink because of your bladder symptoms.

Include beverages in your elimination diet plan to determine which drinks trigger your bladder symptoms.

___

If you feel that your IC symptoms are under control, experiment with different forms of those beverages that still affect you (Example: espresso coffees, herbal coffees, low-acid orange juice, or other flavors of soda).

___

10

Recipes

"The fact is that it takes more than ingredients and technique to cook a good meal. A good cook puts something of himself into the preparation — he cooks with enjoyment, anticipation, spontaneity, and he is willing to experiment."
Pearl Bailey

Preventing Boredom

It does not matter if you are following a weight loss diet, a diabetic diet, or an IC diet, it is easy to get bored and stray off of your meal plan. If you find yourself bored with your food selections while trying to maintain your IC dietary modifications, it is time to experiment!

Trying new recipes can be scary for some IC patients who have finally found some relief with dietary modifications. The trick here is similar to trying new foods in the beginning of an elimination diet:

- Pay attention to individual trigger foods, regardless of the recipe source
- Remember that some trigger foods may not bother you in small quantities

- Try a new recipe only if you feel that your IC symptoms are stable
- To minimize confusion about a recipe's effects on your symptoms, do not try a new recipe if you are also trying another new food, are changing other treatments, or are under stress
- Choose your time to try a new recipe wisely. Make sure that if you stir up your IC symptoms with a new recipe that you have time to recover afterwards
- Keep detailed *Food Intake Diaries* and *Voiding and Pain Diaries* when trying a new recipe to help discern if the recipe affects your IC symptoms

If your IC symptoms are stable, and you are ready to try new recipes, I suggest trying one new recipe per week. Maybe you could designate one particular day, for example, Saturday, as "New Recipe Day." Creating a schedule for experimentation can be less intimidating than staring in a refrigerator wondering what to cook.

Where to Find New Recipes

Almost any cookbook will have some recipes that are safe for you to eat. In fact, many of your family favorites are probably fine as they are, or can be made suitable with only slight modifications of ingredients. If you are ready to try something new, I have included some reputable sources of recipes that can be helpful for IC patients, along with sample recipes to get you started!

The first reference is Beverley Laumann's book, *A Taste of the Good Life: A Cookbook for an Interstitial Cystitis Diet*. Bev Laumann is an IC patient, and has been an IC support group leader for many years in Orange County, California. *A Taste of the Good Life* provides creative recipes and many ideas for recipe modification while at the same time teaching the reader more about IC. Bev is careful to differentiate what we know scientifically about IC and diet, and what we know from observing and talking to IC patients. Purchasing information for *A Taste of the Good Life* can be found in the reference section of this book.

The second reference is the Interstitial Cystitis Network's *IC Chef*, an online cookbook for interstitial cystitis patients (http://www.ic-network.com/icchef/). Started by ICN's Assistant Manager, Diane Manhattan, the *IC Chef* is a collection of recipes submitted by dozens of their members. The cookbook is filled with photographs and provides a wide variety of fabulous recipes for the IC patient to try. Many patients also find help with recipes from other IC patients through the ICN's *Diet and IC Message Board* (http://www.ic-network.com/forum/).

Another place that you may find interesting is the interactive recipe and meal planning website, *Meals For You* (http://www.mealsforyou.com/cgi-bin/home). A nice feature of *Meals For You* is the "Advanced Search" option that you can use to filter recipes by telling the search engine which ingredients to avoid. Although all ingredients that could affect IC are not listed, many such as soy, tomatoes, citrus, chocolate, and caffeine are. Other elements of *Meals For You* include search filters for nutrients, preparation time, and a terrific option that allows you to choose how many servings of a recipe that you want to prepare. With one click, *Meals For You* recalculates the recipe from one up to 300 servings.

And last, another book that I like to recommend is *The Food Allergy Survival Guide* by Vesanto Melina, Jo Stepaniak, and Dina Aronson. This book illustrates how food allergies and sensitivities can affect your symptoms, how to self-assess personal food triggers without compromising nutrition, and how to find hidden sources of problem ingredients in your food. Not all of the recipes contained in this book are suitable for IC patients, but the explanation of how food sensitivities can manifest into physical symptoms makes this book a great asset to any IC patient's reference library. Purchasing information is contained in the reference section of this book.

Finally, conquer dietary boredom by accepting your dietary modifications as a challenge! Experiment with new recipes, modify some familiar ones, and learn to love food again. To get you started, I have included recipes from each of the recommended resources, also including some of my own. All recipes are reprinted or adapted here with permission from the publishers or authors.

From: A Taste of the Good Life:
A Cookbook for an Interstitial Cystitis Diet
by Beverley Laumann

Low-Acid Blueberry "Jam"

The recipe below makes a delicious spread for toast. Not a true jam, it must be kept in the refrigerator.

Ingredients:
- 1/2 c. sugar
- 2 T. flour
- 1 t. Knox unflavored gelatin
- 1/4 t. ground cinnamon
- 2 c. fresh, ripe blueberries
- 1/4 t. lemon extract (optional)
- 6 T. water
-

Thoroughly mix the sugar, flour, gelatin, and cinnamon in a saucepan. Add blueberries, lemon extract and water. Heat while stirring, coating the blueberries with the sugar. Bring to a boil over medium to high heat, stirring continuously to prevent scorching. Continue stirring and cooking one minute more. Pour into a heat-resistant container to cool. Store covered into the refrigerator until ready to use.

Pear-smothered Pork Chops (serves 2)

Ingredients:
- 2 center-cut pork loin chops, about ¾" thick
  1/4 t. ground sage
- Dash salt and pepper
- 1 large, firm-ripe pear
- 2 T. unsulphured molasses
- 2 T. flour
- 1 c. water

In a skillet, brown pork chops in vegetable oil, seasoning with salt and pepper if desired. Remove chops to casserole dish. Sprinkle sage on chops.

Peel and slice pear, placing slices on top of chops. Combine flour with small amount of water to make paste; then add to water. Add molasses to water and mix well. Over low heat, pour liquid into hot skillet, scraping up browned bits of pork. When slightly thickened, pour sauce over chops, cover, and bake at 350° F for 40 minutes, or until done.

Italian Baked Chicken (serves 2)

Ingredients:
- 2 chicken breast halves, skinless
- 1/3 c. unseasoned bread crumbs
- 1/2 t. dried oregano
- 1/4 t. dried marjoram
- 1/8 t. salt
- 1/8 t. pepper
- 1 egg white, slightly whisked
- 3 T. margarine, melted

Rinse and dry chicken. Preheat oven to 375°F. In a bowl, combine breadcrumbs with oregano, marjoram, salt, and pepper. Roll chicken in egg white, then in the crumb mixture to coat. Pour the melted butter in shallow baking dish and turn chicken pieces in it to coat. Arrange pieces in baking dish, not touching, and bake at 375°F until tender, about 50 minutes. Do not turn. Lift out carefully from pan with spatula.

Carrot Salad with Honey Dressing (serves 4)

Ingredients:
- 2 c. grated carrot
- 2 t. fresh mint, finely chopped
- 4 t. dried parsley
- 2 T. raisins (optional)
- 2 t. canola oil
- 1/2 t. ground coriander
- 2 t. honey
- Dash salt

Mix grated carrot, mint, parsley, and raisins, if desired, in a salad bowl. Combine oil, coriander, honey, and salt, whisking together until blended. Pour over salad, tossing to blend. Chill and serve.

Linguine with Clam Sauce (serves 3)

Ingredients:
- 3 cloves garlic, minced
- 1/4 c. olive oil
- 3 cans (6 oz.) chopped clams
- 8 oz. clam juice (bottled)
- 2 T. dried parsley
- 1/2 t. basil
- 1/4 t. salt
- 1/8 t. pepper
- 3 servings of hot, cooked linguine noodles (about 3 c.)

In medium saucepan sauté the garlic in olive oil until tender. Drain chopped clams, reserving liquid from two of the cans. Add reserved liquid, clam juice, parsley, basil, salt, and pepper to the garlic. Bring to boil. Reduce heat and simmer about 5 minutes.

Add chopped clams, heat through, and serve over linguine noodles (or your favorite hot cooked pasta).

Shrimp Variation: Omit one can of chopped clams and substitute ½ c. of tiny cooked cocktail shrimp.

From Interstitial Cystitis Network's IC Chef
http://www.ic-network.com/icchef/

Irish Soda Bread (about 10 servings)
Ingredients:
- 2-1/2 c. whole wheat flour (if tolerated)
- 1 c. all-purpose flour
- 2 T. sugar
- 1-1/2 t. baking soda
- 1 t. salt
- 4 T. butter--room temperature
- 1 egg
- 1-1/4 c. buttermilk--room temperature (if tolerated)

Mix together all the dry ingredients in a large bowl. Using your fingertips, work the butter into the flour mixture until the mixture resembles breadcrumbs. Beat the egg and buttermilk in a separate bowl, and gradually add to the flour mixture. Mix with a spoon at first, and then by hand or mixer when the dough becomes stiff. On a lightly floured work surface, work the dough to thoroughly blend all the ingredients. Do not knead. Sprinkle with flour if the dough should stick. Shape into a round ball and pat the top down slightly, and place on a greased or non-stick baking sheet. Cut a 1/2 in (1 cm) deep cross in the top using a sharp knife or razor blade. Bake in 400°F oven for about 45 minutes, or until it has browned and the cuts have expanded. Remove from oven and cool on a wire rack before slicing.

Scottish Shortbread (serves 30)

Ingredients:
- 2 c. unsalted butter, at room temperature
- 1 3/4 c. powdered (confectioner's) sugar
- 4 1/3 c. flour
- 2 T. granulated sugar (or to taste)

Cream the powdered sugar and the butter, and mix in the flour a little at a time until thoroughly blended. Spread about 1/2 inch (1 cm) thick on a cookie sheet, and prick all over with the tines of a fork. Bake at 300°F for about 30 minutes, until light golden brown. Sprinkle with granulated sugar immediately after removing from oven and allow to cool for 10 minutes before cutting into bars or squares. Allow to cool completely before removing from pan.

Honey Sesame Chicken (serves 4)

Ingredients:
- 4-6 pieces of chicken (thighs are best for this dish)
- 1/2 c. honey
- 1/4 c. sesame seeds
- Salt and freshly ground pepper to taste

Remove the skin from the chicken pieces if you want to reduce the fat content. Season with salt and pepper, and place in a baking pan. A layer of aluminum foil underneath will make clean up easier. Drizzle with honey and sprinkle a liberal amount of sesame seeds on each piece. Bake in a 325°F oven for 30 minutes, or until cooked through.

Egg Drop Chicken (serves 6)

Ingredients:
- 1 lb. pounded chicken cutlets
- 1-1/2 qt. egg drop soup (no MSG)
- 3 c. cooked white rice

Pound chicken cutlets, coat with flour then dip in eggs. Pan fry in pure vegetable oil until cooked through. Pour egg drop soup over chicken and let simmer for 20 minutes. Serve over rice.

Note: You can purchase egg drop soup from your local Chinese restaurant if they do not use MSG or you can make your own:

- 1-1/2 qt. chicken stock
- 2-3 T. cornstarch (to thicken)
- 4-6 eggs

Bring chicken stock to full boil, add cornstarch to thicken, then drop raw eggs one at a time into stock, breaking them up by constantly stirring as they cook.

Tracey's Caramel Candy Bars

Ingredients:
- 1-14 oz. bag of caramels, about 50 pieces
- 1/3 c. milk
- 2 c. flour
- 2 c. quick-cooking or old-fashioned oats
- 1 1/2 c. packed brown sugar
- 1 tsp. baking soda
- 1/2 t. salt
- 1 egg
- 1 c. margarine or butter, softened
- 1 c. chopped walnuts

Preheat oven to 350°F. Grease 9" x 13" baking pan. Heat caramels and milk in a 2 qt. saucepan over low heat, stirring frequently, until smooth. Stir together the flour, oats, brown sugar, baking soda, salt and egg in a large bowl. Stir in butter with fork until mixture is crumbly. Press half of the crumbly mixture in greased pan. Bake 10 minutes. Sprinkle nuts over baked layer. Drizzle with caramel mixture. Sprinkle with remaining crumbly mixture. Bake 20-25 minutes or until golden brown. Cool 30 minutes, loosen edges from sides of pan, and cool completely. For 54 bars cut in 9 rows by 6 rows.

Crunchy Cookies (makes three dozen cookies)

Ingredients:
- 2 c. unsifted flour
- 1 t. baking powder
- 1 t. baking soda
- 1 t. salt
- 1 c. butter
- 1 c. brown sugar
- 1 c. granulated sugar
- 2 eggs
- 2-2/3 c. coconut
- 3 c. corn flake cereal
- 2 t. vanilla

Cream the butter and sugars together. Add the eggs and vanilla and mix well. In a separate bowl, combine the flour with the baking powder, baking soda, and salt. Add the flour mixture to the butter/sugar mixture. Mix well. Lastly, add the corn flake cereal and coconut and mix well. Drop by teaspoonfuls on a greased cookie sheet. Bake at 350°F for 12 minutes. Cookies will look slightly underdone, but they brown a little after being taken from the oven. Make sure you take them from the oven before they look done; in other words, don't bake them until really browned, or they will lose their chewy texture!

Butterscotch Brownies (makes 12 brownies)
Special thanks to Molly

Ingredients:
- 1/4 c. shortening or butter
- 1 c. light brown sugar (packed)
- 1 egg
- 3/4 c. sifted flour
- 1 t. baking powder
- 1/2 t. salt
- 1/2 t. vanilla
- 3/4 c. butterscotch chips

Heat oven to 350°F. Melt butter over low heat. Remove from heat and blend in brown sugar. Cool. Stir in egg and vanilla. In a separate bowl, sift together flour, baking powder and salt. Stir dry mixture into butter, sugar, egg mixture. Fold in butterscotch chips. Spread in well-greased and floured square pan, 8 x 8 x 2. Bake 20-25 minutes until a light touch with finger leaves a slight print. Cut into bars while warm.

Pam's No Bake Cookies (makes 24 cookies)
From Interstitial Cystitis Network member Pam

Ingredients:
- 2 c. sugar
- 1/2 c. evaporated milk (skim evaporated milk is ok)
- 1 stick of butter or low-trans fat margarine
- 3 c. old-fashioned oats
- 1/2 c. peanut butter
- 1 t. vanilla

Heat sugar, milk, and butter, bringing it to a slow boil for 2 minutes. Remove from heat. Stir in oats, peanut butter, and vanilla. Mix thoroughly and drop by teaspoonfuls on wax paper.

Alana's Spinach with Blueberry-Maple Dressing
(serves 4)

Ingredients for Blueberry-Maple Dressing
- 1/4 cup of olive oil
- 1/4 pure maple syrup
- 1/4 blueberries (fresh or frozen)

Put all ingredients into a blender. You can increase or decrease the amount, just keep proportions of ingredients the same. Drizzle over salad below:

Ingredients for Spinach Salad
- 2 c. fresh spinach leaves
- 1 c. fresh blueberries (don't use frozen)
- ½ c. sunflower seeds

Drizzle with Blueberry-Maple Dressing and toss.

From the *Meals For You* website:
www.MealsforYou.com

Blueberry and Pear Cobbler (serves 6)

Ingredients
- 1 lb. canned blueberries
- 1 lb. canned pears, drained
- 1-1/2 cups self-rising flour
- 1/4 cup sugar
- 1/4 lb. margarine or butter
- 1 egg, beaten
- 1/3 cup milk

Drain blueberries, reserving half the syrup. Place pears in a deep pie dish, add the blueberries and syrup. Mix flour and 1/4 c. sugar. Rub in margarine and add enough milk to make a soft dough. Spoon dough over fruit and sprinkle with extra sugar. Bake at 350°F for 35 to 40 minutes, until golden brown. Serve hot, with whipped cream.

Due to the nature of this recipe, MealsForYou.com adjusts the number of servings in multiples of 6 only.

Broiled Pears (serves 4)

Ingredients:
- 4 pears, cut in half lengthwise and cored
- 1 T. plus 1 tsp. water
- 1/4 cup brown sugar
- 1 T. plus 1 t. unsalted butter

Arrange pears in a shallow broiler pan and brush with water. Sprinkle with brown sugar and dot with butter. Turn on broiler. Broil pears for 3-4 minutes or until sugar is bubbly.

Blueberry Pancakes (serves 4)

Ingredients:
- 1 c. all purpose flour
- 1/2 t. baking soda
- 3/4 t. baking powder
- 2 T. sugar
- 1/2 t. salt
- 1 c. buttermilk
- 2 T. vegetable oil
- 1 egg, lightly beaten
- 1 c. blueberries, thawed and drained if frozen

Sift flour, baking soda, baking powder, sugar and salt together in a large bowl. Combine buttermilk, oil, and egg in another bowl. Stir buttermilk mixture into dry ingredients until just combined. Do not over mix. Heat a heavy nonstick skillet or griddle over medium high heat to 375°F. When hot, lightly brush surface with oil. Add about 1/3 c. of batter per pancake to skillet. Sprinkle a few blueberries over each round of pancake batter and cook 2-3 minutes, or until small holes appear in batter and bottom is browned. Turn cakes and cook about 1 minute or until browned. Repeat process until all pancakes are cooked. Serve immediately with desired toppings or keep warm in a 200°F oven until ready to serve.

Due to the nature of this recipe, MealsForYou.com adjusts the number of servings in multiples of 4 only.

Maple Pear Crunch (serves 4)

Ingredients:
- 1/3 cup maple syrup
- 1 T. water
- 4 large ripe firm pears, cored and thinly sliced
- 1/2 c. all purpose flour
- 3 T. yellow cornmeal
- 3 T. brown sugar, packed
- 1/8 t. ground cinnamon
- 1/4 c. unsalted butter, chilled and cut into small pieces

Preheat oven to 375°F. Combine maple syrup and water in a heavy non-reactive saucepan (enamel, anodized aluminum, stainless steel). Cook over low heat 5 minutes or until very hot. Remove from heat. Stir in pear slices and transfer to a buttered baking dish. Set aside. Combine next 4 ingredients in a food processor or bowl. Add butter and cut into dry ingredients until mixture resembles coarse meal. Sprinkle topping over pears and bake 40 minutes, or until bubbly and golden.

Rosemary Beef (for each steak)

Ingredients:
- 1/4 t. rosemary, crumbled or 1/2 t. fresh, minced
- 1/2 t. salt (optional)
- 1 t. pepper
- 1 clove garlic, minced
- 1 strip steak, about 1/4 lb. Each
- 1-1/2 t. olive oil

Prepare grill or broiler. Mash rosemary, salt, pepper, and garlic together in a bowl. Rub mixture into meat and let sit about 15 minutes. Grill meat 3 minutes per side for medium-rare meat; cook longer as desired.

Long Grain Rice with Peas (serves 4)

Ingredients:
- 1 c. chicken stock (no MSG)
- 1 c. water
- 1 c. long grain rice
- Dash of salt (optional)
- 1 1/2c. frozen peas, thawed
- 1 T. unsalted butter or margarine

Combine stock and water in a saucepan over medium high heat. Stir in rice, salt and pepper to taste and bring to a boil. Immediately reduce heat to low. Cover and simmer 15 minutes. Add peas to rice without stirring. Cover and simmer 5 minutes or until rice is tender and liquid is absorbed. Remove from heat and let sit 5 minutes. Add butter and fluff with a fork.

Broccoli with Garlic and Mushrooms (serves 4)

Ingredients:
- 1 oz. butter
- 2 cloves garlic, crushed
- 4 mushrooms, sliced
- 12 oz. broccoli, cut into small florets

Heat butter and garlic in a heavy nonstick pan over medium high heat. Add mushrooms. Cook over medium heat 2 minutes or until tender. Remove from pan, set aside. Add broccoli and stir-fry for 3 or 4 minutes until tender. Return mushrooms to pan, stir until heated through. Serve hot.

Low-Fat Oatmeal Blondies (serves 18)

Ingredients:
- 1 c. all purpose flour
- 1 t. ground ginger
- 1 t. ground cinnamon
- 1/2 t. baking soda
- 1/8 t. ground cloves
- 1-1/2 c. quick cooking oats, uncooked
- 3/4 c. brown sugar, firmly packed
- 3/4 c. pitted dates
- 1/2 c. boiling water
- 1/4 c. unsalted butter
- 1 egg
- 2 egg whites
- 2 t. vanilla extract
- 1 c. powdered sugar, sifted
- 2 T. milk
- 1/2 t. vanilla extract

Preheat oven to 375°F. Sift together first 5 ingredients in a bowl and stir in oats. In a food processor, combine brown sugar and dates. Process until dates are finely chopped. Add boiling water and butter. Process until mixture is smooth. Add egg, egg whites, and vanilla to date mixture. Process to blend. Transfer date mixture to flour mixture. Mix thoroughly by hand. Lightly butter a 9x13 in. baking dish. Transfer mixture to baking dish. Bake 18-20 minutes, or until tester comes out clean when inserted in center. Transfer to a wire rack to cool 5 minutes. Combine powdered sugar, milk and vanilla in a bowl. Mix thoroughly. Spread frosting over bars. Cool completely before serving. Due to the nature of this recipe, MealsForYou.com adjusts the number of servings in multiples of 18 only.

From *Food Allergy Survival Guide*
By Vesanto Melina, Jo Stepaniak, and Dina Aronson

Oven Fries (serves 2 to 4)

These thick, oven-baked french fries are low in fat but resonate with fabulous flavor. Potatoes provide a variety of minerals and are high in vitamin C, even after baking.

Ingredients:
- 2 large russet potatoes
- 1 T. olive oil (optional)
- 1 t. paprika, or 1/2 t. (2 ml) basil
- 1/4 t. salt
- Dash each: pepper, garlic powder, turmeric

Preheat the oven to 450°F. Spray large baking pan with cooking spray and set aside. Scrub the potatoes well and remove any eyes and discolored areas. Peeling is optional.

Cut into wedges or french-fry shapes. Place in a large bowl, sprinkle with the oil, if using, and toss to coat evenly. Sprinkle with the seasonings and toss again so all pieces are evenly coated. Arrange in a single layer on the prepared baking sheet. Bake until golden brown and fork tender, about 30 minutes. For more even browning, turn over once midway through the cooking cycle.

Oven-Roasted Parsnip Fries: Replace the potatoes with 1 pound of parsnips, trimmed, peeled, and cut into french-fry shapes or 1/4-inch-thick diagonal slices.

Rosemary Red Ribbon Rice (Yield: 3 cups)

This rice dish is fragrant, festive, and easy to prepare, making it ideal for everyday meals or for entertaining.

Ingredients:
- 1 1/2 c. vegetable stock or water
- 1/2 c. raisins (preservative free)
- 1 t. crushed garlic
- 1/2 t. salt
- 1/4 to 1/2 t. dried rosemary, well crumbled
- 1 c. white basmati rice
- 1 small red bell pepper, sliced into matchsticks (omit if sensitive to red peppers, many IC patients are not)
- 1/2 c. coarsely chopped walnuts
- 1 T. extra-virgin olive oil

Combine the water, raisins, garlic, salt, and rosemary in a saucepan and bring to a boil. Stir in the rice, cover, and reduce the heat to low. Cook until almost all the liquid has been absorbed, about 18 to 20 minutes.

Remove from the heat, add the bell pepper, walnuts, and oil, and toss gently with a fork until evenly distributed. Cover and let stand for 5 to 10 minutes.

Julie's Favorites

Easy Rice Pudding

Ingredients:
- 4 c. cooked rice (can be left over from meal)
- 1 egg
- 1/2 c. skim milk
- 1 t. vanilla
- 3/4 c. sugar
- 1/2 t. cinnamon (if tolerated)

Break egg into medium bowl and beat until smooth. Add milk and vanilla, continue beating. Combine rice, sugar, (cinnamon) and liquid ingredients in medium saucepan. Continuously stir ingredients over medium heat, simmering for 5 minutes. Be careful not to burn. Remove from heat. Pudding can be enjoyed warm or cold!

Blueberry Muffins

Ingredients:
- 1/2 c. butter, softened
- 1 c. sugar
- 2 eggs
- 2 c. flour
- 2 t. baking powder
- 1/2 t. salt
- 1/2 c. evaporated milk
- 1 t. vanilla
- 2 c. fresh blueberries

Preheat oven to 350°F. Cream butter and sugar. Add eggs and mix well. Add flour, baking powder, salt, milk and vanilla. Fold in fruit. Pile high in muffin tins. Bake 25-30 minutes.

Blueberry Breakfast Casserole (serves 8)

Ingredients:
- 12 slices homemade-type white bread
- 8 oz. cream cheese, cubed
- 1 c. fresh blueberries
- 12 large eggs
- 1/3 c. maple syrup (may omit)
- 2 c. milk

Sauce Ingredients:
- 1 c. sugar
- 2 T. corn starch
- 1 c. water
- 1 c. fresh blueberries
- 1 T. unsalted butter

Prepare the night before: Remove crusts from bread and cube bread into 1-inch slices. Layer ingredients in a buttered 9 x 13-inch glass baking dish:

1. Half of the bread cubes (the bottom)
2. Cubed cream cheese
3. Blueberries
4. Other half of the bread cubes

In large bowl, whisk together eggs, syrup and milk. Pour over bread mix, cover, and chill over night.

In the morning: Preheat over to 350°F. Cover casserole with foil. Bake for 45-55 minutes or remove when puffy and golden brown.

For blueberry sauce: Stir sugar, cornstarch, and water in small saucepan. Cook mixture over medium heat for 5 minutes, stirring frequently. Mixture will thicken. Stir in blueberries and simmer the mixture, stirring frequently, about 10 minutes or until berries have "burst." Add butter and stir the sauce until butter is melted. Serve casserole with sauce.

Imitation Cream Soup (for casseroles or soup base)

Ingredients:
- 12 oz. can of skim evaporated milk
- 2 T. butter or margarine
- 2 T. flour
- 1/2 t. salt
- 1/4. t. garlic powder
- 1 T. onion chopped fine (or use chopped chives if you are sensitive to onion)
- 1/4 t. pepper (if tolerated)

Melt butter in medium saucepan over medium heat. Add flour blending with wisk until smooth. Slowly add milk, wisking constantly until mixture thickens, remove from heat. Blend in seasonings.

Use instead of canned cream soups in recipes:
- **Simple soup:** Add mushrooms, celery or chicken, 1 c. skim milk
- **Casserole:** Add 1 c. chopped chicken or tuna, vegetables and 3 cups noodles. Bake at 350°F for 20 minutes
- **Hearty Soup:** Add 1 c. chicken, 1 1/2 c. skim milk, 2 cubed potatoes, 2 diced carrots, 1/2 c. peas, and 1 stalk chopped celery. Simmer over medium heat until vegetables are cooked through.
- **Quick White Pizza:** Put 2-3 T. of sauce on a pita. Add strips of baked or grilled chicken, mushrooms, sprinkle with basil, top with mozzarella cheese and bake until bubbly!

Butternut Squash

Ingredients:
- 1 butternut squash (may use acorn squash)
- 1/4 c. butter or margarine
- 1/3 c. brown sugar
- dash (1/4 t.) salt

Peel and cube squash. In medium saucepan, combine squash and enough water to cover plus 2 inches. Heat to a boil, cooking until very soft. Remove from heat, drain off water, and mash. Add butter, brown sugar, and salt. Bake at 350°F for 20 minutes.

Taking Control

Using your personal "OK" list, look for one or two new recipes to try each week. You can try a new recipe or rework one of your own. Try designating one day of the week to try new recipes!

11

Dietary Supplements for IC

"Medicine and quackery have always been close, if not compatible, partners. At times, they may appear to have separated, but sooner or later, in one place or another, they wind up reunited."
Varro E. Tyler in *The Honest Herbal*

Important Legal Stuff

Any discussion of complementary and alternative medicine (CAM) is certain to stir some controversy; therefore, I introduce this topic cautiously. The information presented here is not medical advice. Treatment of interstitial cystitis is highly individualized. Drug interactions are becoming more common as people have access to more over-the-counter medications and alternative options for treatments. Individual patients may have co-existing conditions that could be complicated by the use of "natural" treatments. No recommendations for use or dosages are provided or implied below. I strongly urge you to contact your physician for information regarding any change you wish to make in your lifestyle.

Some Quick Definitions:

The National Center for Complementary and Alternative Medicine (NCCAM): An entity of the National Institutes of Health (NIH), NCCAM is the federal government's lead agency for scientific research on Complementary and Alternative Medicine (CAM). NCCAM is dedicated to exploring complementary and alternative healing practices in the context of rigorous science, training CAM researchers, and disseminating authoritative information to the public and professionals.

Conventional Medicine: Conventional medicine is medicine as practiced by holders of M.D. (medical doctor) or D.O. (doctor of osteopathy) degrees and by their allied health professionals, such as physical therapists, psychologists, and registered nurses. Some conventional medical practitioners also practice CAM.

Complementary and Alternative Medicine (CAM): A group of diverse medical and health care systems, practices, and products that are not presently considered to be part of conventional medicine." *Complementary* medicine is used together with conventional medicine. *Alternative* medicine is used in place of conventional medicine. Some scientific evidence may exist regarding individual CAM therapies, but often there are still critical questions concerning safety and effectiveness of CAM therapies. *Integrative medicine* combines conventional medical therapies and CAM therapies.

Categories of CAM: The five domains of CAM recognized by NCCAM are:

- Alternative Medical Systems
- Mind-Body Interventions
- Biologically Based Therapies
- Manipulative and Body-Based Methods
- Energy Therapies.

This chapter on CAM and IC will focus on Biologically Based Therapies including dietary supplements, and herbal products.

Dietary Supplements: The Dietary Supplement Health and Education Act (DSHEA), which Congress passed in 1994, defines dietary supplements as a substance (other than tobacco) that is taken by mouth, contains one or more dietary ingredients (vitamins, minerals, herbs, amino acids, etc.), and is labeled as being a dietary supplement. Whether a substance is classified as a dietary supplement, conventional food, or drug is based on its intended use. Dietary supplements may not advertise to diagnose, cure, mitigate, treat, or prevent a disease. The Food and Drug Administration (FDA) is the agency responsible for regulation of DSHEA regulations.

Buyer Beware

It is important to mention here that dietary supplement ingredients sold in the United States before October 15, 1994 are not required to be reviewed by FDA for their safety before they are marketed, because they are assumed to be safe for use in humans based on their usage history. Incidentally, the FDA does not regulate the quality and standardization of dietary supplements. Some supplement producers voluntarily follow Good Manufacturing Practice (GMP) regulations that define how dietary supplements must be prepared, packed, and stored.

Also, due to the scarcity of high-quality research for most dietary supplements, it is critical that you check with your physician before taking any dietary or "natural" substance for your IC or any other health condition. Many products have ingredients that could interfere with your conventional medications or therapies, and just as important, your experience with a product can help educate your physician about CAM options. In other words, if something is helping (or hurting) you, that information might help your physician help other patients in the future.

Locating Quality Dietary Supplement Information

Selling dietary supplements and related products is a multi-billion dollar industry. People with chronic illnesses, chronic pain, or terminal illnesses are the most vulnerable consumers, wanting to believe that something can cure them, or relieve their pain. It is wise, therefore, to be an educated consumer concerning any medical treatment (alternative or conventional) you may want to try. Just because something is printed or broadcast doesn't make the information true. Take the time to investigate any scientific studies that have been done regarding therapies and treatments, especially questioning safety and effectiveness of the treatment. When reading about research results, be aware of such details as:

- When the study was done—nutrition information is evolving constantly as researchers refine their methods
- The number of people in the study—results of studies using small subject groups are not always applicable to a larger universal group
- The study design—double blind studies using a control group are the gold standard
- The researchers' credentials—look for PhD's, physicians, dietitians, nurses, and food scientists
- The identification of funding (NIH studies and other independent foundations)—critically examine studies sponsored by an organization that has a special interest in the outcome.
- The comparison of the research with parallel research—do the results of the study complement other information on the same topic? If not, is contradictory information discussed?

You can find an abundance of information about supplements on the Internet. Unfortunately, the information you find must be carefully and critically evaluated. Good places to start looking for information are the NCCAM website at http://nccam.nih.gov/ and at http://quackwatch.com. Discuss any information that you find with your medical care team.

A Sampler of Dietary Supplements

In this section you will find information about various dietary and botanical supplements occasionally mentioned in reference to IC treatment. This information is compiled from the NIH Office of Dietary Supplements and a variety of other sources. Although care has been taken to provide accurate and factual information, due to the nature of the topic, no recommendations for use or dosages are provided or implied below. I strongly urge you to carefully evaluate any information that you get regarding health and wellness.

Acid Reducers

Acid reducers include products whose action neutralizes some of the acid in foods and oral antacid agents, either prescription or over the counter (OTC). Many patients report successful reduction of symptoms when using acid reducers. Prelief and pHControl are both OTC products that you can add to food or take orally. Various brands of oral antacids can also be effective in reducing the symptoms of IC patients.

Acidophilus

Acidophilus is often recommended by alternative practitioners to maintain normal intestinal bacteria levels if you have taken, or are taking, antibiotics. Opportunistic yeast infections can be a concern for some IC patients due to the number of antibiotics they may have taken over time.

Aloe Vera

Aloe vera has been touted as a miracle plant in folklore for centuries. According to the Desert Harvest Aloe website, aloe vera aids in tissue repair and acts as an antibiotic, pain reliever, and anti-inflammatory agent. Aloe is also rich in vitamins, minerals, and essential elements. Desert Harvest has sponsored double blind placebo controlled clinical trials of their patented aloe product in IC patients with "incredible" results. Aloe vera is reported to have an extremely low incidence of side effects.

Chondroitin Sulfate

The American Academy of Orthopaedic Surgeons states that chondroitin sulfate is a natural substance found in the body that prevents other body enzymes from degrading the building blocks of joint cartilage. Chondroitin is also a component of connective tissues—holding muscles, nerves, and blood vessels together, and may also act as an anti-inflammatory agent. There is emerging evidence to suggest that chondroitin sulfate acts as a bladder coating. Chondroitin sulfate is found in Algonot's CystoProtek and ProstaProtek, combined with olive kernel oil for increased absorption. People with shellfish allergies should not take products with chondroitin sulfate.

Essential Fatty Acids

Essential fatty acids are fats that the human body requires to function properly. Essential fatty acids cannot be synthesized by the body from other fatty acids and must be obtained from food. Essential fatty acids are essential in cell membrane development and repair. Low levels of essential fatty acids may increase cardiovascular disease risk.

Fiber

Fiber is the part of fruits, vegetables, and grains that the body cannot digest. Soluble fiber dissolves easily in water and takes on a soft, gel-like texture in the intestines. Insoluble fiber passes through the intestines almost unchanged. The bulk and soft texture of fiber help prevent hard, dry stools that are difficult to pass. Constipation can increase inflammation in the pelvic region, thus increasing IC symptoms. Diets high in fiber may help reduce the risk of cardiovascular disease and some forms of cancer.

Garlic

Garlic has been shown to have small but significant effects on reducing cardiovascular disease. Garlic also has been shown to have some anti-inflammatory and antiseptic effects in animal and human studies. The one side effect of garlic, and garlic supplements is a garlic odor, which may, or may not be reduced by using special preparations.

Glucosamine Sulfate

A key ingredient in the formation of joint cartilage, glucosamine sulfate is also present in the soft material between bones and joints and has mild anti-inflammatory abilities. Side effects are few, but some people may be allergic to glucosamine sulfate. CystoProtek contains glucosamine sulfate.

L-Arginine

L-arginine is a vital amino acid present in protein. L-arginine is a semi-essential amino acid, meaning that in normal circumstances the body can produce enough of the amino acid for its needs. Supplementation of L-arginine has shown promising, but mixed results. L-arginine improves nitrogen balance and protects proteins from breaking down and may also increase the effectiveness of some cancer treatments. Research is continuing. Potential side effects include nausea, abdominal cramps, and diarrhea.

Multivitamins

Multivitamins and highly fortified foods often cause an IC patient's bladder to flare. Culprits here include excess vitamins that are excreted in the urine, artificial coloring, and fillers. If you are concerned about your nutrition, try taking a children's formula vitamin without artificial colors or flavors.

Quercetin

Some of the most compelling research done using nutrition supplements in urological disorders involves quercetin. Quercetin is a constituent of plants that seems to have many medicinal purposes. Quercetin is a natural anti-inflammatory agent, and has been investigated for use in IC and chronic prostatitis with promising results. CystaQ, CystoProteck, and ProstaProtek all have quercetin as a component of their product. Clinical trials involving quercetin are ongoing.

Vitamin C (Ester C)

Many IC patients are concerned that they are not consuming enough vitamin C because they are avoiding citrus fruits. It is easy to meet your body's vitamin C requirements, however, by eating a selection of other fruits and vegetables including blueberries, winter squash, broccoli, cabbage, and potatoes. Vitamin C supplements are a common bladder irritant, however, some patients do well with Ester C, a low-acid version of vitamin C.

Taking Control

What types of complementary or alternative medicine treatments have you used in the past?

_____
_____
_____
_____
_____
_____
_____
_____
_____

What were your experiences with these treatments? (Were they helpful or not? How did they help?)

_____
_____
_____
_____
_____

What types of dietary supplements have you taken in the past? For what conditions?

_____
_____
_____
_____
_____

Where did you get your information about the dietary supplements that you tried? Did you talk to your physician about taking supplements?

_____
_____
_____
_____
_____

What dietary supplements are you taking now, especially those that you take for IC?

_____
_____
_____
_____
_____

Did you talk to your physician about them before you tried them? If not, have you talked to him or her since then to let them know if the dietary supplements are helping you or not?

_____
_____
_____
_____
_____
_____
_____
_____
_____
_____

12

Exercise and Fitness

> *"All parts of the body which have a function, if used in moderation and exercised in labours in which each is accustomed, become thereby healthy, well-developed and age more slowly, but if unused and left idle they become liable to disease, defective in growth, and age quickly."*
> Hippocrates, the Father of Medicine

Making Fitness a Priority

Imagine that! Nearly 1700 years ago, Hippocrates recognized that exercise is an essential component of a healthy lifestyle. Unfortunately, physical activity is not often a priority when you are first diagnosed with a chronic illness like IC. Pain, fatigue, and unpredictable urinary frequency can seem like impossible barriers to maintaining an active lifestyle. Physical discomfort from bike seats, chlorinated pools, and wet swimsuits can be problems as well.

Nevertheless, being diagnosed with IC should not get in the way of you caring for the rest of your body. We all know that extended periods of inactivity can raise your risk of cardiovascular disease, various cancers, diabetes, and obesity. In addition to combating these health issues, an active lifestyle lowers the risk of depression and is simply more fun! You might have to modify your approach as you pursue the activities you enjoy. Just as eating well with the IC diet has required you to do some planning, staying active with IC will require the same. The great news is that these adjustments are all manageable.

What is Fitness?

Fitness is a collection of physical attributes that measure the amount and type of physical activity that your body can do. These physical attributes include:

- Cardiorespiratory endurance: The heart and lungs' ability to get oxygen to the muscles for sustained activity
- Muscular endurance: The ability of the muscles to sustain activity without fatigue
- Muscular strength: The force exerted by a muscle during an activity
- Body composition: The percentages of lean muscle and adipose tissue (fat) in the body
- Flexibility: The range of motion for joints in the body

Each of these attributes is important for overall health. Luckily, many exercises target several of these attributes at one time. Walking, biking, dancing, and swimming all combine cardiorespiratory endurance and muscular endurance. In the long term, they improve body composition. Swimming, yoga, and some forms of dancing improve overall flexibility. Weight training improves both body composition and muscular strength. Ultimately, you should participate in a wide variety of activities to maintain overall fitness.

How Much Exercise Do I Need?

It is important to ask your physician how much exercise he or she recommends, especially if you have been inactive for longer than a few weeks. Keep in mind that exercise does not mean you have to take aerobic classes or joining a running club. You do not even need to do all of your exercise at one time. A reasonable goal is to do more physical activity today than you did yesterday. You might start by walking 20 minutes each day over your lunch hour, gradually increasing the time to 30 minutes each day. It is the collective activity that makes a difference in your fitness level.

Pedometers are a good way to gently challenge yourself to get moving. These simple devices clip to the pocket of your pants or your waistband and count the number of steps that you take in a day. Some pedometers will measure miles or count calories, but all you really need to know is the number of steps you take each day. Most health authorities say that 10,000 steps a day is a good goal. Ideally, you should be able to take 2500 steps in 20 minutes, which is approximately one mile.

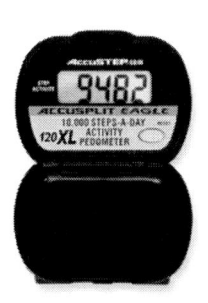

Before the idea of walking roughly four miles per day scares you away, keep in mind that a pedometer accumulates ALL of your daily activity. If you spend time walking your dog, shopping, or gardening, all of those steps "count" toward your total for the day. Again, I suggest that you just do a little more each day until you get there (or beyond). Everyone starts somewhere. Checking your pedometer frequently can become a fun way of challenging yourself. You may even find yourself taking the stairs instead of the elevator or walking to the store just to take more steps!

You can find pedometers at sporting goods stores, department stores, and even pharmacies. A reliable online source with a generous guarantee is Accusplit (www.Accusplit.com), the same company that makes stopwatches and timers for professional sporting events. Each Accusplit pedometer comes with a "leash" which prevents the pedometer from hitting the floor if it becomes detached from your pocket (Easy to do in the restroom!). You will also want to remember to remove your pedometer from your waistband before throwing your pants in the laundry. My editor has had several close calls that way!

Levels of Intensity

Low intensity activities take longer to burn the same number of calories as higher intensity activities. If you have been inactive, or you are having a low-energy day, you can do light activities like simple yard work, housecleaning, shopping, or cooking. A person should be able to sing while doing a light intensity activity.

Medium intensity activities include walking (15 minute/mile), biking, dancing, weeding, digging a garden, carrying groceries into the house, or carrying baskets of laundry upstairs. A person should be able to hold a conversation while performing moderately intense activity.

Higher intensity activities would include fast walking (10 minute/mile) or walking with a load uphill, heavy manual labor, playing basketball, stair climbing, or hiking over uneven and hilly paths. Generally, these activities are performed for several minutes at a time, alternating with more moderately intense activity. In any case, if you become winded, short of breath, or can't carry on a conversation, the activity is too strenuous for your current fitness level. If this happens, reduce the intensity of the exercise.

Measuring Intensity

Once you become serious about challenging your fitness level, you might consider monitoring your heart rate while exercising. Some people buy simple heart rate monitors for this, but it is easy to take your own pulse:

Taking Your Heart Rate

You can take your pulse at the neck, the wrist, or the chest. We recommend the wrist. You can feel the radial pulse on the artery of the wrist in line with the thumb.

Place the tips of the index and middle fingers over the artery and press lightly. Do not use the thumb.

Take a full 60-second count of the heartbeats, or count for 30 seconds and multiply by 2. Start the count on a beat, which is counted as "zero."

You can use your heart rate to determine how intensely you should be working during exercise. The basic guidelines regarding your heart rate are based on your age and fitness level. Keeping your heart rate within this "target zone" ensures that you are working out at maximum efficiency. Keeping an eye on your target zone not only keeps you from taking things too easy, but also helps you avoid needless overexertion.

Determining your target zone is pretty straightforward. For moderately intense physical activity, a person's target heart rate should be 50% to 70% of his or her maximum heart rate. This maximum rate is based on the person's age:

> **Doing the Math**
>
> An estimate of your maximum age-related heart rate can be obtained by subtracting your age from 220.
>
> For example, for a 50-year-old person, the estimated maximum age-related heart rate would be calculated as 220 - 50 years = 170 beats per minute (bpm).
>
> The 50% and 70% levels would be:
> - 50% level: 170 x 0.50 = 85 bpm, and
> - 70% level: 170 x 0.70 = 119 bpm
>
> Thus, moderate-intensity physical activity for a 50-year-old person will require that the heart rate remain between 85 and 119 bpm during physical activity.

Once you are comfortable with moderately intense exercise levels, discuss with your doctor the possibility of pursuing higher-intensity exercise. For higher-intensity activities, your target heart rate should be 70% to 85% of your maximum heart rate. This is calculated using the same formula as used above, substituting "70% and 80%" for "50% and 70%." (Centers for Disease Control, 2005)

Activity with IC

With some creativity and an occasional modification, IC patients can stay physically active in their daily lives. In addition to increasing your daily activity at work and at home, you can walk stairs if you cannot get to a gym, do stretching or yoga, dance to music, or use a treadmill while watching TV.

If walking too far from home makes you anxious, walking in shopping malls can be a fantastic alternative. You are close to bathrooms, and you do not have to depend on good weather. Or, you can break a long walk up into three different segments. I walk a mile circuit in my neighborhood two or three times, knowing that I will pass by my home every ten minutes in case the "urge" hits me. Also, some IC patients wear bladder control pads while they exercise for a little added security.

Riding a bike poses some different challenges for IC patients. Not only can the pressure of the seat be uncomfortable, but a ride over rough terrain can be jolting to your bladder. Mountain bikes can be a wonderful solution to both problems. Shop carefully for a bike that has high quality shocks on each of the wheels and the seat, and opt for a wider saddle seat. You might also consider upgrading to a seat that is especially designed for the anatomy, sporting a hollow middle. Or, if you are looking for a biking activity that you can do in your home or at the gym, try a recumbent bike! Always check with your physician or physical therapist if you have pelvic floor problems before you ride a bike.

In addition to walking and biking, consider going for a swim. Some IC patients experience an increase in symptoms when they swim. Yet swimming can be an excellent low impact activity for people whose bladders seem to bother them with every step. Once again, modification is the rule. If you have your own pool, ask your pool supply company about sanitation chemicals that don't use chlorine, or switch to an ozone purification system, which reduces the amount of chlorination necessary. If you do swim in a chlorinated pool, keep your time in the water short, and rinse off after you get out. Whenever you swim, you should change into dry clothes immediately to avoid the discomfort cause by lounging in wet swimsuits.

No matter what you do, it is important to have fun. To combat boredom (and increase overall fitness), participate in a variety of activities. If you are interested in trying yoga or taking dance classes, check with your local adult education department. These classes are usually reasonably priced and require a limited obligation. Getting to meet new people is a great bonus!

Preventing Injuries

Many common injuries associated with physical activity can be avoided by following these few sensible guidelines:
- Check with your physician before you start any new exercise program. Some treatments and medications can alter your tolerance to different activities
- Warm up your muscles by slowly increasing the intensity of the activity
- If you are just beginning an exercise program, take it easy at first, gradually increasing time and intensity
- Drink a small glass of water before you begin your activity, sipping on more water during the time that you remain active
- Vary your activities to prevent boredom and overuse of any individual muscle group
- Use appropriate equipment, shoes, and clothing for the activity
- Listen to your body—monitor your level of fatigue, heart rate, and physical discomfort. Breathlessness and muscle soreness could be danger signs
- Be aware of the warning signs and signals of a heart attack, such as sweating, chest and arm pain, dizziness, and lightheadedness
- Cool down as you finish the activity—decrease the intensity gradually and stretch the muscles used for the activity

Taking Control:

How has IC affected your activity level?

What activities are you willing to try?

What are your overall fitness goals?

Use your journal to record your daily activities.

13

Making Peace with Stress

"I believe that a simple and unassuming manner of life is best for everyone, best both for the body and the mind."
Albert Einstein

What is Stress?

Despite all of the psychological talk these days about stress, many people are still not sure what it means. For example, stress itself is neither negative nor positive. Instead, it is our reaction to stress that turns stress into "distress." Most IC patients learn early that stress can aggravate their symptoms. Please understand that this is not the same as saying that your symptoms are all in your head. Stress, more exactly the body's response to stress, produces chemical and physical changes that cause our bodies to react in ways that are intended to protect us, but they can also cause damage to our bodies.

The first thing to keep in mind is that stress can be either "external" or "internal." Examples of external or physical stress include loud noises, extreme heat or cold, malnutrition, injuries, illnesses, toxins, travel, heavy labor, exercise, harsh weather, smoking, and drug or alcohol use. Internal stress can include emotions like anger, resentment, envy, revenge, tension, anxiety, excitement, guilt, fear, rejection, failure, success, depression, love, joy, expectations, boredom, and even frustration. If you are surprised about the "positive" emotions being listed there, consider the stress people experience when planning weddings or building their dream house!

Fight or Flight

Imagine that a fire spontaneously breaks out in a store where you are shopping. Some of the people around will call 911. Some will work to fight the fire. Of course, some will flee, or run from the scene. The body's physical responses to this stressful situation (the "fight or flight" response) include:

- Increased release of stress hormones—frequently triggering IC symptoms
- Surges of blood sugar released—providing quick energy for muscle and brain functions
- Accelerated heart rate, increased respiration, and increased blood pressure—improving the flow of oxygen and energy to the muscles and brain
- Increased cholesterol levels—providing a sustained form of energy
- Increased blood clotting ability—preparing the body to heal potential wounds from "fighting"
- Increased sweating—keeping the body cool during "battle"
- Dilation of pupils—maximizing vision
- Slowed digestion—allowing the body to "focus" on the stressful event

Although all of these physical reactions are valuable when a fire breaks out, many times the stressful events we experience do not require the same level of physical activity that fighting a fire demands. For example, when you are subjected to pressure at work, it is unlikely that you will physically have a fight with your boss. Or, if you are in a traffic jam, you probably are not going to get out of your car and start running. Yet, in each case, your body goes through all of those physiological and chemical changes of stress.

This unmanaged stress negatively affects body systems. Nutrition resources are depleted rapidly. The risk for heart disease and stroke increases. Headaches and muscle aches are more common in people under stress. Both men and women can experience fertility problems, and the body is more susceptible to illness (cancer, infection, colds, and flu) because of a weakened immune system.

Many health problems are stress related. People under stress are more susceptible to ulcers and irritable bowel disease. Bingeing behavior can increase after a stressful episode, making weight management difficult. On top of that, stress hormones encourage fat to be stored. Finally, as most IC patients know, unmanaged stress can cause an increase in urinary symptoms.

Thankfully, by managing your stress, you can decrease the negative effects on your body. Learn to recognize when stress is affecting you and practice methods to deal with it:

- Take action if you can—procrastinating on a project or sweeping problems under the rug only increases stress in the long run

- Commit to a healthy diet—a healthy diet not only keeps the body from going into stress related to malnutrition, but it also reestablishes nutritional balance when nutrients are depleted, and fortifies the immune system

- Exercise—exercising gives the body something *physical* to do when it is in a state of stress and reduces the effects of stress by using up the chemicals released in the "fight or flight" phenomenon

- Avoid the temptation to "relax" by using alcohol or drugs when under stress—these substances only increase stress on a body

- Practice deep breathing, yoga, massage, meditation, or prayer; hug someone; get a pet—giving your body permission to relax when a situation is beyond your control lessens the impact of stress on your body

- Talk to someone, call a friend, write your congressman, make an appointment with your clergyman or a therapist, even write a letter to yourself about the stress—many times once we give words to our troubles, they do not seem as overwhelming as we originally thought they were

- Forgive those who have hurt you and forgive yourself for not being perfect—acceptance is a great stress moderator

- Enjoy a hobby, take up a craft, or take a class and learn something new—feeling a sense of accomplishment can raise your spirits, especially if you have unending problems at work

- Let go when there is nothing you can do—putting your problems behind you is much healthier than obsessing about problems that can never be solved

Emotions and Interstitial Cystitis

What about times when stress doesn't seem to be the cause of your personal distress? Many times IC patients will comment on how emotional they get. Others will notice an increase in anxiety and/or depression as they struggle with their disease and its various symptoms. Maybe your family has commented that you lose your temper more often, or you find you cannot tolerate what others consider a normal amount of noise or chaos around you.

Certainly, having a chronic illness is life changing, and a fair amount of emotion would be considered normal as you struggle to get a diagnosis, experiment with treatments, and navigate through the stages of acceptance (denial, anger, bargaining, and acceptance). However, other things that contribute to mood disturbances may not be so obvious.

First, the cardinal symptoms of IC (pain, frequency of urination, and unrelenting urinary urgency) are enough to put anyone into a state of anxiety or depression. For those who spent years searching for a diagnosis, including those whose family or physician told them that their angry bladder was a psychological disorder, the imprinting of anxiety when symptoms flare can be even more pronounced. In other words, your body subconsciously and habitually goes into a state of anxiety when you flare because that is all it knew to do before you learned other coping techniques.

Anxiety can also be exaggerated by the unpredictability of flares, uncertainty of how certain foods will affect you, or simply being somewhere new and not knowing where the bathroom is located. In fact, when I asked other IC patients for ideas on what to include in *Confident Choices*, the most common suggestion was to tell people what to eat when they are in a flare. As simple as that concept may seem, most of us just cannot think straight when we are in a flare, and we can benefit from any direction that others can give us. Thus, I added a chapter on "Food for Flares."

You may be surprised at some other, hidden reasons that you have mood changes when you have IC. Many medications have side-effects that affect the emotional center of the brain. Some act as depressants, and others may increase anxiety. In addition to the medications, the nervous system for the lower pelvis is connected near the part of the brain where emotions are generated. As the nerves send those frantic messages of pain and urgency, the emotional part of the brain can also be stimulated making it seem like a mood change comes out of nowhere. In a similar body-mind connection, when we are under stress, the body releases hormones that can wreak havoc on an already tender bladder.

So now that we know why we feel emotional at times, what can we do about it? First, if you suspect that medications may be causing you trouble or that you may need medical help to calm your emotional issues, please seek the help of your doctor. Second, remember the stress reduction techniques discussed previously in this chapter. Take three deep breaths, find a quiet place and pray or meditate, do some simple stretching exercises, or just take a walk. Third, cut out sugar and caffeine to reduce the chemical effects that can aggravate your moods. (Hopefully by now, you don't drink caffeine anyway, right?) Lastly, try to understand and forgive yourself. As you learn to recognize the various causes of mood disruptions in your own body, you will gain better control of your life overall.

Sleep and Stress

Although it may seem impossible to many people who have IC, it is essential that you get sufficient rest. In 2004, psychologist David Dinges, PhD, of the University of Pennsylvania School of Medicine reported that, on average, more than 60 percent of Americans sleep less than seven hours per night and the same percentage have problems sleeping at least a few nights each week. Yet seven to eight hours of good quality sleep is essential for health, safety, productivity and overall well-being. Sleep deprivation can also intensify physiological stress, which can affect the quality of sleep, often leading to a vicious cycle.

Now, it is not always easy to convince a healthy person to make sleep a priority, so how is a person with IC supposed to get the required amount (and quality) of sleep? To be honest, I am not sure I have the answer to that question. I just know you have to keep trying. During the first couple of years after I was diagnosed with IC, I went to the doctor a half dozen times looking for a reason why I was so exhausted. After making sure there wasn't any underlying cause for the fatigue, my doctor said to me gently, "Julie, maybe you are just one of those people who needs to take a nap now and then."

There it was; I had permission to rest, and now I am passing that permission on to you. The bottom line is that IC is tiring. Frequent urination and pain can make long periods of sleep very difficult. When we don't get enough quality sleep we are not able to function well, affecting nearly all of our waking hours. The best we can do is rest when we need to, as often as we can. Take some extra time to relax before bedtime, settling on a nightly routine, if possible. Wear earplugs or run a fan for white noise to muffle random noises that could wake you unnecessarily. Some patients find relief from using the stick on heating pads used for menstrual cramps. Others find that a warm bath can help them relax and get a longer period of uninterrupted sleep. If, after trying some of the self-help methods for getting better sleep, you still cannot get enough sleep, please don't hesitate to talk to your physician. You might find that one of the common medications for IC can actually help you sleep better, or maybe there is another medical reason for your fatigue. Of course, maybe you are just one of those people who needs to take a nap now and then.

Taking Control:

How does stress affect your IC symptoms?

What techniques do you use to help manage stress in your life?

In what ways can you improve your ability to manage the effects of stress?

Do emotions affect your ability to cope with your disease? If so, how?

In what ways can you improve your ability to manage the effects of emotions on your body?

_____
_____
_____
_____
_____
_____

Does your IC interrupt your sleep? In what ways can you improve your sleep patterns?

_____
_____
_____
_____
_____
_____

14

IC Diet Success Stories

"The most beautiful people we have known are those who have known defeat, known suffering, known struggle, known loss, and have found their way out of the depths. These persons have an appreciation, a sensitivity, and an understanding of life that fills them with compassions, gentleness, and a deep loving concern. Beautiful people do not just happen."
Elizabeth Kubler-Ross in *On Death and Dying*

Does Diet Help?

Determining your individual trigger foods can be a long and tedious process, and many of you probably want to know if dietary modification is worth the effort. Until we get more research on diet and IC, there is no better way to illustrate the effects that dietary changes can have on IC symptoms than to talk to other patients.

I asked fellow IC patients to share with you their diet modification success stories. I also asked what steps they took to determine their problem foods. What follows is a sampling of their responses.

Donna

At the time my IC was diagnosed (1975), not much thought had been given to a diet connection. When I had my first hydrodistention, I was encouraged to drink lots of juices, especially cranberry, and I was given cranberry juice mixed with 7-up in the hospital. It took me a while, but I did figure out that juices brought on pain for me, so I stopped drinking juices. The next trigger I discovered was coffee. A friend who doesn't have IC suggested that I try not drinking coffee to see if it helped.

It did take me a long time, but I finally discovered my other trigger foods. And when IC diets came out, all of my triggers were listed there. It would have been much, much easier for me if I could have had access to those lists from the beginning.

We still have a long way to go in treating IC, but in the past thirty years we have also come a long way.

Sharon

When I was finally diagnosed with IC, my urologist told me there was nothing he could do for me. He said, "Go home and deal with it." So, I had to find my own way. I realized that certain things caused me more pain, like juice, jelly, and even my own tap water. I quickly figured out that acid was a problem, yet I was still in pain.

I surfed the Web and found the wonderful ICN website about 6 years ago. I have been "hanging around" ever since. I learned from the food list that this diet involved more than just avoiding acidic foods. I started following the diet, and slowly without the help of any medicines, I started to gain control over my life again.

I tried another urologist. Because I walked into his office so in control of my symptoms, he refused to believe I had IC, he wouldn't even test me. He said, "Don't let anyone ever tell you, you have IC, it will ruin your life."

Today, I still control my pain mostly through diet. I only take a small amount of medicine at bedtime. Other medicines I have tried have not agreed with me. Looking back, I'm glad I was forced to take control of my IC to start with. It makes me feel like I have more control over it (IC), than it does over me.

Jolene

Donna and I were both diagnosed at about the same time, in 1975. I was just 16 at the time, and she is right, diet was not talked about a lot then. In fact, I didn't have a name for my illness until years later when I got my medical records. I was told I had an ulcer-like condition in my bladder, and that I would most likely need more silver nitrate instillations to help.

I really started putting two and two together about diet sometime in the '80's. I think I saw an article that Vicki Ratner (of the Interstitial Cystitis Association) had written about IC. I knew as soon as I saw that article that (IC) was what I had. She mentioned a little about diet in that article. It was the first real information I heard about foods affecting IC. My diagnosing urologist had said to watch spicy stuff, but not a whole lot more was mentioned that I recall.

After taking away the trigger foods, it didn't take long to see that they were indeed a problem. That is also how I know *now* when I have eaten something I shouldn't have, because of how my bladder reacts. After you have been on the diet for a while, your bladder lets you know.

Alexa

I definitely benefited from modifying my diet. After I was diagnosed I did the elimination diet, starting with plain chicken, steamed broccoli, and plain white rice. Gradually (over a period of months) I phased in various foods. It was tedious, but I'm still benefiting today from taking the time to do it 8 years ago. I believe that avoiding my trigger foods, in combination with some medications, has been the key to my success in treating my IC symptoms.

Annie

I guess I have always known that what a person consumes does affect the bladder, even for healthy people. Before IC, I had bladder infections every few years (not regularly....just one every 3-4 years). I always felt better when I drank cranberry juice when I had an infection.

When my IC began, that is how I knew something "different" (not just an infection) was going on. I drank cranberry juice and I felt worse, not better, so I cut it out. I was drinking a cola every day and noticed that I felt better if I switched to root beer instead of cola. Then a doctor suggested I might have IC. I had heard of IC but knew very little about it. What I did know was that there was no cure.

Right away I wondered about a connection between my diet and the severity of my symptoms. I started searching the Internet and found the ICN. I looked for diet information first thing and, of course, found it in the Patient Handbook. Well, I had fits when I saw the extent of the IC Diet! I wasn't diagnosed yet and, though I had that "gut feeling" that IC was what I was experiencing, I went into denial. I didn't want to believe it was happening to me! And that diet thing…NO WAY could that many things be affecting me! Yes, I understood diet could affect anyone's bladder, but surely no one was that sensitive to all of those foods and additives!

I wasn't getting any relief from my symptoms and finally decided I'd better go back and look at the diet list again. Ughh!!!!!! Not only no more cola, but also no other sodas, no tea, not even decaf, no chocolate, no tomato sauces…etc.! No way could I give up all that! So I reasoned, ok…I'll limit just the top 5 offenders.... certainly that would be enough sacrifice to take care of it. Of course, I didn't get much better and, still in denial, made the big rationalization that I was one of the few who wasn't very diet sensitive.

Eventually, I reached that desperate point when I was ready to try anything to get relief. I printed out several copies of the diet, clipped one on my fridge, put one in my purse and kept another on the kitchen table. I went shopping and burst into tears in the grocery store when I realized how much I had to avoid. I was desperate, however, and I stuck to buying only things from the "Usually OK" column of the diet. I pledged to give it a two-week honest try. It was incredibly hard, but I did it. I was feeling a bit better so I pledged to stick with it another two weeks. After that time I was feeling much better and started to realize just how much help I was getting from carefully following the diet. With time, and trial and error, I found that I was actually extremely diet sensitive and could control much of my pain and reduce my frequency with diet alone. It took finding the right meds to add to the diet to get me to a better place, but diet is key to maintaining control of my IC.

Now, when I see a newly diagnosed ICer submit a question on the ICN message boards, stating they don't really think diet is helping them, I just want to reach out and hug them. I understand exactly where they are in the process of accepting the IC Diet. It's incredibly difficult. It does get easier once we get past that initial denial and find how much it can help most of us. I still despise the fact I must avoid so many favorite foods and beverages. But I have learned that following my diet is my choice. I can feel pretty good, or I can give into that craving for chocolate and have to deal with the pain of making that decision. Most of the time the pain price is not one I am willing to pay.

Amaris

I'd thought I'd give the IC diet thing a try since it was something I could immediately do and control. I posted a copy of the IC food list on the fridge and gave a copy to my hubby, since he usually does the grocery shopping. The first month I strictly stuck to the "Usually OK" list. Gradually, I began trying food from the "May Be OK" list and the "Usually Not OK" list. I kept a small journal in my purse at all times so that I could make notes of what foods caused trouble a couple of hours later. I also began using Prelief, which was helpful especially when going out to eat. Also, one of the first things we did was to get a water filter (we'd been without for a couple of months, and I suspect that the city water was significantly contributing to the constant pain since I drink a lot of water).

Keeping a journal was the most helpful tool for me to determine what my trigger foods are. I would make a list of a couple new foods I'd like to try and meticulously try them one by one in small doses and at least twice. This was a great help at work because I could figure out what specific menu items I could and couldn't order from the local cafeteria/restaurants. It was extremely helpful in figuring out that certain preservatives and artificial sweeteners were triggers, "hidden" in those long lists of ingredients. Plus, I didn't have to go around remembering which foods were OK, since I had them written down!

I still miss alcohol and key lime pie, among other things, but once you experience pain free days and weeks, eating trigger foods is just not worth it!

I believe that it's the combination of diet and meds that have helped me feel better. I still adhere to the list of foods I've found that are safe, although I can occasionally stray and eat something like lasagna with Prelief and not experience a flare—something I clearly couldn't do a year ago.

The other added bonus of my IC diet is that Hubby and I eat even healthier than before. Between his love of cooking, and mine of baking, there are very few things we can't make for ourselves, which gives me complete control over what ingredients we use.

Jenny

I think I see some improvement from diet alone; however, it took a few weeks to notice. It seems to take me a few "transgressions" before it really catches up to me. So for me, I think it's a build-up effect. However, when I first thought I *might* have IC, cutting out the cranberry pills I had been taking for my "bladder infection" helped immensely.

Vicki

I had been taking those cranberry pills too. Nasty, nasty! But I thought I was dealing with some on-going infection, and was told the cranberry pills would help!

When diagnosed with IC, my urologist gave me a (short) list of foods to avoid. His office also pointed me towards ICN, where I've learned so much from other patients. I guess I tend to be a bit obsessive. When I learned that diet could actually make me feel better, but that not everyone reacts to the same foods, I immediately went on a chicken, potato, peas, or corn diet to find my trigger foods (all cooked from scratch, so I had control of additives). On Sunday, I would bake a couple of chickens for the family dinner and put the leftovers in small packages in the freezer. I'd fix a variety of meals for my family throughout the week, but microwave my IC frozen dinner for myself. Within a week, I was already feeling so much better and really empowered! I had some control over this!

Originally I'd planned to do this for two weeks before adding new foods, but by day eleven I needed variety! I began to add foods from the "Usually OK" list, one at a time. If my bladder threw a fit, I'd go back to my "safe" diet until I felt fine, and then try that (trigger) food one more time. I had to make sure it was truly that specific food item and not a fluke. As a food passed the test, my "safe" diet expanded.

Eleven months have passed, and so far the foods and additives I've found I must avoid make up a pretty short list -

although some of my favorite things are on it, like tomatoes! I have learned that Prelief does allow me to indulge in limited portions of most of my known trigger foods. I still treat all new food items with suspicion, trying small amounts and hoping for the best! I don't trust my bladder to any restaurant personnel. I am always taking Prelief before dining out, even if the food seems like it'll be safe. But I must admit, sometimes even though I know better, occasionally I think, "Just one small taste will probably be okay." DUH! The pain puts me back on the straight and narrow for another couple of months!

Kadi

One thing I did that was super helpful was to print out a copy of the *IC Food List* from ICN and post it on the fridge. I ate only from the left hand column (the "Usually OK" list) and marked down each time something caused a spike in my symptoms. Eventually, I started gingerly trying things in the middle column (the "Maybe OK" list) with Prelief, again marking down OK, NOT OK, or OK in small quantity with Prelief. This list has been super helpful in explaining the diet to my dad (who LOVES to cook for people, especially those he loves) and a dietitian, who helped me develop balanced meal plans and taught me to cook in a more time-efficient way.

I can say that I enjoy food again (even though I am very strict in following the diet), because I think it's one of the reasons I can still work and don't need much in the way of painkillers.

Stacey

Okay, I'm sort of new to the diet thing. My whole life I've known that there are certain things that will bother my bladder. When I was a kid, I couldn't drink any soda with caffeine or any fruit juices. I also couldn't eat super acidic fruit like oranges. When I was sort of re-diagnosed with IC at age 23, two years ago, I figured it would be the same things that have always bothered me. Though I looked through the diet, I didn't give it much thought.

After about two years with no treatment working, I finally decided maybe there was something else I was eating that was bothering me. I started by giving up my morning bowl of cereal. I didn't see much change. Then I reached a breaking point. My husband went online and did some research on diet with me. We decided I ought to at least give it a try. That was about two and a half months ago. I started with giving up everything in the "Usually Problematic" column. Within a week or two, I started feeling better. I decided after the New Year to do the elimination diet and see what exactly bothers me.

I started the elimination diet, and it was a very rocky start for me. Then we had an ice storm and lost power, so I have gotten sidetracked, but I'm going to get back on track. I went to the urologist last week and was told for the first time that my urine was pretty clear. I didn't have any sort of inflammation like I usually do. That was encouraging to me.

I still dread having to do this. I think it stinks, but after my appointment and also after reading some of these notes from other patients, I am much more encouraged. I have sat here reading them this evening with tears in my eyes. I feel like I may be able to get my life back more to normal. Of course, if it is my diet, I am going to be a bit angry with myself that it took me so long to realize it, but I can't change the past. I can only make a difference for the future.

Taking Control

IC is a disease about coping and managing lifestyle activities such as exercise and diet. When patients share their stories two people are helped. Not only is the person hearing or reading the story helped by learning from another person's experience, but also the storyteller often experiences a step toward acceptance and healing. As you come to the end of this book, what would you like to tell other IC patients? What is your IC diet modification story?

15

Resources

Organizations

Confident Choices
P.O. Box 210086
Auburn Hills, MI 48321
Web address:
http://www.NutraConsults.com/confidentchoices.html
Email: NutraConsults@aol.com
Phone: 248-961-3613

I established Confident Choices, a nutrition education company, to educate patients and medical professionals about the unique nutritional needs of interstitial cystitis patients.

Highlights of Confident Choices:
- Individual and group nutrition and lifestyle counseling exclusively for IC patients by a registered dietitian who specializes in IC
- Options for consultation include traditional office visits, home visits, and phone consultations
- Support group workshops about IC dietary modification, lifestyle strategies and supplement education

- Continuing education workshops for registered dietitians
- A monthly newsletter dedicated to providing IC dietary support, resources, and reviews of research.
- The IC Shop Online, interfacing with ICN's IC Shop and Amazon.com to provide purchasing options for IC food and comfort products as well as educational resources

Interstitial Cystitis Network (ICN)
PO Box 2159
Healdsburg CA 95448
Web address: http://www.ic-network.com
IC Shop Sales: 707-433-0413
Patient Help Line: 707-538-9442
Fax: 707-538-9444

ICN is a publishing company dedicated to interstitial cystitis and other pelvic pain disorders. They strive to present the world's best research, information, and support directly into the homes and offices of their users (patients, providers & IC researchers).

Highlights of the ICN website:
- A comprehensive online patient handbook, which outlines treatments, dietary concerns, research, physician locator, coping strategies, and more
- A free email magazine, and subscriber supported magazines and special reports
- An extraordinary message board system monitored by dozens of volunteers, dedicated to providing online emotional support and valid medical information regarding IC, treatments, and coping strategies
- The IC Shop and Market, offering food, beverages, supplements, and comfort products as well as resource publications
- Numerous resources for dietary modification including the "IC Chef" and "Fresh Tastes by Bev"

- "Meet the IC Expert" guest lectures given as online, moderated chats, with transcripts of lectures cataloged in the Patient Handbook

Interstitial Cystitis Association (ICA)
110 North Washington Street
Suite 340
Rockville, MD 20850
Web Address: http://www.ichelp.org

E-mail: icamail@ichelp.org
Telephone: 301-610-5300
Toll-free: 800-HELP ICA

The Interstitial Cystitis Association (ICA) is a national 501(c)(3) nonprofit organization. The ICA is dedicated to educating the medical community and the public about IC. They provide support and information for IC patients and their loved ones via their Website, newsletters, publications,, as well as a network of National Patient Support Advocates, and IC Connections telephone and email lists. The ICA works to promote and provide research funding, to find effective treatments, and a cure for IC.

Highlights of the ICA:
- Various publications and resources available for IC patients, their families, and healthcare professionals
- Physician education references
- Current research summaries
- Physician registry
- Quarterly newsletters for both Patients and Healthcare Professionals, as well as a monthly online news digest
- Regional and National Forums and Conferences on IC for both Patients and Healthcare Professionals
- Continuing political advocacy efforts for IC research funding at the Federal level

American Dietetic Association
120 South Riverside Plaza, Suite 2000
Chicago, IL 60606-6995
Web address: http://www.eatright.org
Telephone: 800-877-1600

ADA is the world's largest organization of food and nutrition professionals, with nearly 65,000 members. The ADA website has a search feature called "Find a Nutrition Professional" to help you locate a registered dietitian near you.

Other Websites

Meals For You
http://www.mealsforyou.com

Meals For You is operated by Point of Choice, a leader in online recipes and nutrition. The Meals For You website provides users with recipes, meal plans, nutrition information, newsletters, and shopping lists, using their proprietary database of over 10,000 recipes. *Meals For You* offers an "Advanced Search" option, where a user can filter recipes by telling the search engine which ingredients to avoid.

WeGoShop.com
http://www.wegoshop.com/

WeGoShop.com is the largest, nationally expanding, full-service, personalized grocery shopping and home delivery company in the United States. By using the WeGoShop.com grocery delivery service, you can avoid impulse shopping and unwanted trips to fast food restaurants and convenience stores. There are absolutely no mark-ups on your grocery items. You pay the same amount that the grocery store of your choice charges for the groceries you order, including sale and "club card" prices, plus the modest grocery shopping and delivery charge.

National Institutes of Health
National Institute of Diabetes and Digestive and Kidney Diseases
http://kidney.niddk.nih.gov/kudiseases/pubs/interstitialcystitis

A US government sponsored website containing valuable information about diagnosis, causes, treatments, and research opportunities for interstitial cystitis.

Nutrition.gov
Web address: http://www.nutrition.gov

An extensive US government sponsored website providing nutrition information.

Information contained on Nutrition.gov:
- Dietary Supplements
- Diseases and Disorders
- Food Allergies
- Food Composition
- Food and Nutrition Assistance
- Food Safety
- Nutrition Recommendations
- Shopping, Cooking & Meal Planning
- Sports & Exercise
- Weight Control

US Department of Health and Human Services
Healthy People 2010
Web address: http://www.healthypeople.gov

Healthy People 2010 is a government sponsored, health promotion and disease prevention challenge for individuals, communities, and professionals. *Healthy People 2010* identifies a wide range of public health priorities. The Website provides guidelines and educational materials.

US Department of Health and Human Services
National Institutes of Health
National Center for Complementary and Alternative Medicine
Web address: http://nccam.nih.gov/

The National Center for Complementary and Alternative Medicine (NCCAM) is one of the 27 institutes and centers that make up the National Institutes of Health (NIH). The NIH is one of eight agencies under the Public Health Service (PHS) in the Department of Health and Human Services (DHHS).

NCCAM is dedicated to exploring complementary and alternative healing practices in the context of rigorous science, training complementary and alternative medicine (CAM) researchers, and disseminating authoritative information to the public and professionals

Quackwatch.com
Web address: http://www.quackwatch.com

Quackwatch.com is dedicated to providing balanced information and research on questionable CAM practices, aiding consumers as they make educated decisions about their health care.

FitDay.com
Web address: http://www.fitday.com

FitDay is an online diet and fitness journal. This website is comprehensive, colorful, and fun to use. Users track their food intake, exercises, weight loss, and goals online. FitDay provides feedback and analysis that helps users stay on track with their diet and fitness goals.

Books

A Taste of the Good Life: A Cookbook for an Interstitial Cystitis Diet
by Beverley Laumann
Publisher: Freeman Family Trust Publications (July 1, 1998)
ISBN: 096657060X

A Taste of the Good Life is a wonderful reference on IC and diet, rich with recipes and includes substitutions for people on multiple dietary restrictions.

The Interstitial Cystitis Survival Guide: Your Guide to the Latest Treatment Options and Coping Strategies
by Robert M. Moldwin
Publisher: New Harbinger Publications (October 30, 2000)
ISBN: 1572242108

Dr. Moldwin, a highly regarded urologist who specializes in IC, has taken the mystery out of IC diagnosis, treatments, and related conditions in this easy to read, comprehensive guide for physicians and patients about interstitial cystitis. This book includes a section dedicated to men who suffer from interstitial cystitis, a discussion of pelvic floor dysfunction, and even a chapter about pregnancy and IC.

Patient to Patient: Managing Interstitial Cystitis and Overlapping Conditions
by Gaye Grissom Sandler, Andrew B. Sandler
Publisher: Bon Ange LLC; 1st edition (February 1, 2001)
ISBN: 0970559003

Patient to Patient is generously written from the hearts, minds, education, and most of all, personal experiences of this husband and wife team. Gaye, an IC patient and Aston-Patterning movement and muscle re-education specialist, and Andrew, a health administration expert with a degree in psychology, offer patients their unique perspective when discussing common problems that IC patients and their loved ones face.

A Headache in the Pelvis: A New Understanding and Treatment For Prostatitis and Chronic Pelvic Pain Syndromes
by David Wise
Publisher: National Center for Pelvic Pain; 3rd Rev Edition (March 15, 2005)
ISBN: 0972775528

A Headache in the Pelvis describes the details of the Stanford Protocol, a treatment for prostatitis and other chronic pelvic pain syndromes that was developed at Stanford University Medical Center in the Department of Urology. This book may be helpful for both men and women who live with the frustrating and sometimes disabling symptoms of pelvic dysfunction such as: pain, difficulty with urination or sexual problems.

When the Body Says No
by Gabor Mate
Publisher: Wiley; 1st edition (April 11, 2003)
ISBN: 0471219827

When the Body Says No carefully illustrates the connection between a person's health and their emotional state. Anyone who suffers from an autoimmune disease, an inflammatory condition, or cancer will find this book valuable. Gabor Mate develops a persuasive argument for the importance of understanding stress and its connection to disease.

Celebrate Life: New Attitudes for Living with Chronic Illness
by Kathleen Lewis, RN, MS, CMP, LPC
Publisher: Arthritis Foundation (October 25, 1999)
ISBN: 0912423242

Lewis, diagnosed with lupus, fibromyalgia, and osteoarthritis, is a medical psychotherapist and licensed counselor who celebrates her life with chronic illness and helps others do the same through her counseling services and writing. *Celebrate Life* provides a rich collection of strategies ranging from including how you can advocate for yourself with medical professionals, how to reward yourself, and how to find the way along the path to acceptance of living with chronic illnesses.

Food Allergy Survival Guide: Surviving and Thriving With Food Allergies and Sensitivities
by Vesanto Melina, Dina Aronson, Jo Stepaniak
Publisher: Healthy Living Publications (August 1, 2004)
ISBN: 157067163X

Enjoy life and food again. Written by three registered dietitians, *The Food Allergy Survival Guide* is yet another fantastic guide when dealing with food allergies and sensitivities. Readers can learn how food allergies and sensitivities affect their bodies, how to self-assess personal food triggers without compromising nutrition, and learn how to find hidden sources of problem ingredients in their food. This book also contains vegetarian meal planning suggestions.

IC & Pain: Taking Control
Publisher: The Interstitial Cystitis Association
Ordering info: 1-800-HELP ICA or www.ichelp.org

This 100-plus-page paperback book is the first book dedicated exclusively to a thorough discussion of the pain issues unique to IC patients, and it is a wonderful resource for every IC patient and healthcare provider.

IC & Pain: Taking Control includes chapters on Pain Basics, The Treatment of Pain, Chronic Pain Issues and Challenges, and Getting Help. This unique book reflects the most up-to-date thinking from renowned IC experts on how to manage IC pain successfully, including a special section of patient questions answered directly by leading IC clinicians and researchers.

Nutritional Supplement Information

Information regarding these dietary supplements is taken directly from the individual company's marketing materials. Inclusion in this publication does not constitute endorsement, nor does exclusion from this list imply lack of endorsement.

Desert Harvest Aloe
1140 Amstel Drive
Colorado Springs, Colorado 80907
Toll Free: 800-222-3901
Fax: 719-598-8918
E-mail: support@desertharvest.com
Web address: http://www.desertharvest.com

Desert Harvest whole-leaf aloe vera capsules are unique. Their aloe vera plants are grown organically, using no pesticides or chemical fertilizers. The leaves are harvested and cold processed to preserve the active ingredients. Desert Harvest does not use preservatives, artificial ingredients, or additives. The aloin and aloe emodin (chemicals that cause diarrhea) are removed using a patented formula. Aloe vera works as an antibiotic, pain reliever, anti-inflammatory, and promotes tissue regeneration.

Desert Harvest was the first aloe vera company that discovered the connection between whole leaf aloe and IC. They sponsored the first double-blind, placebo-controlled clinical trial of aloe vera use in IC patients, and have two more studies planned.

Prelief

AkPharma Inc.
PO Box 111
Pleasantville, NJ 08232
Toll Free: 800-994-4711
E-mail: prbetty@akpharma.com
Web address: http://www.akpharma.com

Prelief is an acid reducer made from calcium glycerophosphate, a dietary supplement. IC patients have used Prelief successfully for years. In retrospective studies, Prelief helped to reduce bladder pain associated with consuming high acid foods in 70% of IC patients, and reduced urinary frequency in over 60% of patients. Clinical studies are in progress to document Prelief's effectiveness.

CystoProtek

Algonot
5053 Ocean Boulevard
PO Box 294
Sarasota FL, 34242
Toll Free: 800-ALGONOT (800-254-6668)
E-mail: feedback@algonot.com
Web address: http://www.algonot.com

Algonot researchers have found that CystoProtek, a unique natural formula of chondroitin sulfate, glucosamine, quercetin, sodium hyaluronate and olive kernel extract, can help relieve many of the symptoms associated with cystitis and interstitial cystitis. CystoProtek has the anti-inflammatory power of chondroitin sulfate and quercetin but also includes, glucosamine sulfate, and sodium hyaluronate to help heal the damaged bladder.

CystoProtek is the result of years of research into interstitial cystitis by Theoharis Theoharides, MD, PhD. Dr. Theoharides is a professor of Pharmacology, Internal Medicine and Bio Chemistry at Tuft's University in Boston. Algonot, LLC is a corporation dedicated to combining scientific investigation with natural healing. An outstanding team of prominent physicians and scientists from Ivy League universities form its advisory board.

CystaQ
Farr Laboratories
11100 Santa Monica Blvd. #560
Los Angeles, CA 90025
Toll Free: 877-284-3976
E-mail: service@cystaq.com
Web address: http://www.cystaq.com

CystaQ is a dietary supplement that was specifically developed to help patients with interstitial cystitis. CystaQ's ingredients include a proprietary formula of quercetin, bromalain, papain, cranberry powder, black cohosh (root) skullcap, wood betony (leaf), passionflower, and valerian.

pH Control
pH Sciences, Inc.
P.O. Box 65260
17230 12th Ave NE
Seattle, WA 98155
Toll-free: 877-363-2243
In Seattle: 206-364-6761
Fax: 206-364-5369
Email: info@phsciences.com
Web address: http://www.phsciences.com

The pH Control Alka-Plex compound is formed into a tablet specifically designed to pass through the stomach without dissolving. pH Control delivers an effective, natural, and safe acid neutralizer into the intestinal tract where it can be absorbed into the body fluids and be carried into the bladder and urinary tract. The effectiveness of pH Control has been proven in laboratory testing and pre-clinical studies. More studies are underway.